Multiple
Choice
Questions in

PLASTIC
SURGERY

Kayvan Shokrollahi

Iain S Whitaker

Hamish L~

Foreword by Robert M. Goldwy~

tfm Publishing Limited, Castle Hill Barns, Harley, Nr Shrewsbury, SY5 6LX, UK. Tel: +44 (0)1952 510061; Fax: +44 (0)1952 510192 E-mail: nikki@tfmpublishing.com; Web site: www.tfmpublishing.com

Design & Typesetting: Nikki Bramhill BSc Hons Dip Law
First Edition: © September 2009
ISBN: 978 1 903378 66 3

Cover images:
Left: © 2009 Kayvan Shokrollahi BSc MB ChB MSc LLM MRCS (Eng) FRCS (Plast)
Middle and right: © 2009 Welsh Centre for Burns and Plastic Surgery, ABM NHS Trust.

ii

Printed by Gutenberg Press Ltd., Gudja Road, Tarxien, PLA 19, Malta. Tel: +356 21897037; Fax: +356 21800069.

Contents

iii

Page

iv

Foreword

The editors, contributors and publisher of this book have achieved their objectives of "covering the breadth of plastic and reconstructive surgery including burns" with their choice of subjects and questions, the clarity of their answers and the pertinence of their references. Any reader interested in what we do or think we do will find this book an excellent experience in learning. It is not a potpourri of facts to be digested and disgorged in order to pass an examination. It is Continuing Medical Education the way it was intended.

Most who will be consulting this book will be preparing for an examination. I remember the unpleasantness associated with what I then considered a stressful intrusion into my already overfilled life. Like my patients, however, who had to undergo surgery to continue their lives, I had to endure these exams to continue my career. My advice then to myself and now to you who may be in a similar situation is not to fight the process. Convert the nuisance, if you regard it as such, into an opportunity to be a more knowledgeable, better doctor. Admittedly information is not the same as wisdom but neither is it a deterrent.

Many of those required to take a written examination have asked me why is it necessary in this era of instant retrieval of information to still store so much data in their heads? A good question. Those who ask it are seldom satisfied with the likely predicted answer that knowing as many facts as possible will provide more quickly a sturdier and wider platform on which to build intellectually and professionally.

Let us not forget that it is more important how we perform as a doctor - as a plastic surgeon with a patient - than at a credentialing session. One needs, however, the formal imprimatur.

In a multiple choice question that has more parts than Caesar said did Gaul, one has an unusual, if not necessarily wanted, opportunity to think about a problem from several angles, thereby enlarging one's horizon beyond what it would have been with a single answer question: yes or no? Socrates well understood this principle.

Hopefully this book will help the reader consolidate what he or she already knows and will stimulate creativity and spur scientific advance.

The American economist and social critic Thorstein B. Veblen (1857-1929) stated: "The outcome of any serious research can only be to make two questions where one question grew before." (*Evolution of the Scientific Point of View*, 1908).

Again my congratulations to the editors and contributors for so effectively and pleasantly enlarging our knowledge and perspective of the broad range of our specialty and its potential.

Robert M. Goldwyn MD
Clinical Professor of Surgery
Harvard Medical School, Boston, Massachusetts
Editor Emeritus, *Plastic and Reconstructive Surgery*
Former Member of the American Board of Plastic Surgery

Who doesn't love a quiz, especially one you can conduct alone and where the answers are immediately available? Quizzes can serve as learning aids, knowledge testers, as reassurance or as a spur to further study. They can be a check of currency for one's own knowledge as well as a test for those revising for exams. But most of all, they are fun.

This collection of tests of plastic surgery knowledge is well ordered, well structured and most of all enjoyable. This is plastic surgery in note form, only turned around from the dreary litany of fact to the much more engaging challenge: "Did you know that....". I will be surprised if it does not gain a very wide audience, not only among those preparing (in whatever country) for the exit exam in plastic surgery, but also amongst trainers, established surgeons and anyone curious about the level of their own knowledge. It also stands as monument to the extraordinary scope of our specialty, and anyone who knows most of this will know most of the depth and breadth of the specialty, as defined by a wide range of contributors from many nations and many areas of subspecialisation. I value it highly and hope others will too.

Professor Simon Kay BA, BM, BCh, FRCS (Plast), FRCSE (Hon)
Consultant Plastic Surgeon, Leeds Teaching Hospitals, UK
Professor of Hand Surgery, University of Leeds
Past President, British Society for Surgery of the Hand
President, British Association of Plastic,
Reconstructive and Aesthetic Surgeons

Contributors

AMERICA

Pejman Aflaki MD
Research Fellow, Division of Plastic Surgery, Brigham and Women's
Hospital, Harvard Medical School, Boston, Massachusetts

**Professor Ian T Jackson MBChB, MD(G) (Hon), DSc (Hon), FACS,
FRCS (Ed), FRCS(C) (Hon), FRCS(G)(Hon), FRACS (Hon)**
Director, Craniofacial Institute, Southfield, Michigan
Editor-in-chief, *European Journal of Plastic Surgery*

Professor William C Lineaweaver MD, FACS
Rankin Plastic Surgery Center, Brandon, Mississippi
Editor-in-chief, *Annals of Plastic Surgery*

Maurice Nahabedian MD, FACS
Department of Plastic Surgery, Georgetown University Hospital,
Washington DC

Professor Foad Nahai MD, FACS
Paces Plastic Surgery, Atlanta, Georgia
Clinical Professor of Plastic Surgery, Emory University
President, International Society for Aesthetic Plastic Surgery (ISAPS)
Past President, American Society for Aesthetic Plastic Surgery (ASAPS)
Editor-in-chief, *Aesthetic Surgery Journal*

Bohdan Pomahac MD
Assistant Professor in Surgery, Harvard Medical School
Medical Director, Brigham and Women's Hospital Burn Center, Boston,
Massachusetts

Luis Scheker MD
Associate Clinical Professor of Surgery (Plastic and Reconstructive), University of Louisville, Louisville, Kentucky
Assistant Consulting Professor of Surgery at Duke University
Plastic, Reconstructive and Hand Surgeon, Kleinert, Kutz and Associates Hand Care Center, Louisville, Kentucky

ARGENTINA

Braulio Peralta MD
Assistant Professor, Plastic Surgery Unit, Pontificia Universidad Catolica Argentina (UCA), Buenos Aires

AUSTRALIA

Damien Grinsell MBBS, FRACS
Royal Melbourne and St Vincent's Hospitals, Melbourne

James Katsaros FRACS
Director of The Department of Plastic and Reconstructive Surgery, Royal Adelaide Hospital, Adelaide

Warren M Rozen MBBS, BMedSc, PGDipSurgAnat, PhD
Jack Brockhoff Reconstructive Plastic Surgery Research Unit, Melbourne

BELGIUM

Professor Phillip N Blondeel MD, PhD, FCCP
Professor of Plastic and Reconstructive Surgery, Department of Plastic and Reconstructive Surgery, University Hospital Gent, Gent

Professor Moustapha Hamdi MD, PhD, FCCP
Professor of Plastic and Reconstructive Surgery, Department of Plastic and Reconstructive Surgery, University Hospital Gent, Gent

CANADA

Professor Stefan O P Hofer MD, PhD, FRCS(C)
Wharton Chair in Reconstructive Plastic Surgery
Chief Division of Plastic Surgery, Department of Surgery and Department of Surgical Oncology, University Health Network, University of Toronto, Ontario

HONG KONG

Professor Andrew Burd MD, FRCS(Ed), FCSHK, FHKAM(Surg)
Chief of Division of Plastic and Reconstructive Surgery, Department of Surgery, The Chinese University of Hong Kong, Prince of Wales Hospital, Shatin, SAR
Editor-in-chief, *Journal of Plastic, Reconstructive and Aesthetic Surgery* (JPRAS)

HUNGARY

Norbert Nemeth MD, PhD
Assistant Professor, Vice-Chair, Department of Operative Techniques and Surgical Research, Medical and Health Science Center, University of Debrecen
Secretary General of the International Society for Experimental Microsurgery (ISEM)

INDIA

Shobha Chamania MS
Choithram Burns Unit and Research Centre, Indore
Director, Interburns (India)

ITALY

Professor Paolo Santoni-Rugiu MD, PhD
Formerly Professor of Plastic Surgery, S. Chiara University Hospital, Pisa
Past President of the European Association of Plastic Surgeons (EURAPS)

NETHERLANDS

Professor Moshe Kon MD, PhD
Head of Department, Plastic, Reconstructive and Hand Surgery, University Medical Center, Utrecht
Secretary General, European Association of Plastic Surgeons (EURAPS)

NEW ZEALAND

Professor Swee T Tan MBBS, FRACS, PhD
Professor in Plastic Surgery, University of Otago; Consultant Plastic & Cranio-Maxillofacial Surgeon and Director of Surgery, Hutt Valley DHB, Wellington.

PAKISTAN

Shariq Ali FRCS
Director of Karachi Burns Centre, Civil Hospital and Dow University of Health Sciences, Karachi
Director, Interburns (Pakistan)

SINGAPORE

Tan Kok Chai MBBS, FRCS (Eng), FAMS
Associate Professor, Plastic and Reconstructive Surgery, Chairman of Division, Singapore General Hospital, Singapore

Colin Song MBBCh, FRCS (Edin), FAMS
Associate Professor, Head and Senior Consultant Plastic Reconstructive and Aesthetic Surgery, Department of Plastic Reconstructive & Aesthetic Surgery, Singapore General Hospital, Singapore
Director, Postgraduate Medical Institute, Singapore General Hospital, Singapore

SLOVENIA

Zora Janzekovic
Vinarska, Maribor

SWEDEN

Rafael Acosta MD, EBOPras
Consultant Plastic Surgeon, Chief Reconstructive Microsurgery Section, Department of Plastic Surgery, University Hospital Uppsala, Uppsala

TAIWAN

Professor Fu-Chan Wei MD, FACS
Professor of Plastic and Reconstructive Surgery, Chang Gung Memorial Hospital and Dean of the College of Medicine at Chang Gung University

UNITED KINGDOM

Dean Boyce MD, FRCS, FRCS (Ed), FRCS (Plast)
Consultant Plastic and Hand Surgeon, Welsh Centre for Burns and Plastic Surgery, Morriston Hospital, Swansea, Wales.
Training Programme Director and Regional Specialist Advisor for Plastic Surgery in Wales

David Gault MB ChB, FRCS
Consultant Plastic Surgeon, London Centre for Ear Reconstruction, The Portland Hospital, London

Henk Giele MBBS, MS, FRCS, FRACS (Plast)
Plastic, Reconstructive and Hand Surgeon, Lead Clinician, Department of Plastic, Reconstructive and Hand Surgery, Oxford Radcliffe Hospital, Oxford

Hamish Laing MBBS, BSc, FRCS (Plast)
Consultant Plastic Surgeon, Welsh Centre for Burns and Plastic Surgery, Morriston Hospital, Swansea, Wales
Communications Officer of the British Association of Plastic, Reconstructive and Aesthetic Surgeons (BAPRAS)

Tom Potokar MBChB, DA (UK), DTM&H, FRCS (Ed), FRCS (Plast)
Consultant Plastic and Burns Surgeon, Welsh Centre for Burns and Plastic Surgery, Morriston Hospital, Swansea, Wales
Founder and Director, Interburns

Awf A Quaba FRCS (Plast)
Honorary Consultant Plastic Surgeon, St Johns Hospital, Livingston

Donald Sammut LRCP, MRCS, FRCS (Plast)
Consultant Hand Surgeon, The Hand Clinic, Windsor and King Edward VII Hospital, London
Senior Consultant and Lecturer, Istituto Clinico Humanitas, Milan, Italy

Taimur Shoaib MD, FRCS (Plast)
Consultant Plastic Surgeon, Canniesburn Plastic Surgery Unit, Glasgow Royal Infirmary, Glasgow

Kayvan Shokrollahi BSc, MB ChB, MSc, LLM, MRCS (Eng), FRCS (Plast)
Specialist Registrar in Burns and Plastic Surgery, Welsh Centre for Burns and Plastic Surgery, Morriston Hospital, Swansea, Wales

Philip J Sykes OBE, MA, FRCS
Formerly Consultant Plastic Surgeon, Welsh Centre for Burns and Plastic Surgery, Morriston Hospital, Swansea, Wales
Past President of the British Association of Plastic Surgeons

Christopher G Wallace BSc (Hons), MBChB, MRCS, MS
Specialist Registrar in Burns and Plastic Surgery, Department of Plastic Surgery, Wythenshawe Hospital, Manchester. Formerly, Microsurgical Clinical and Research Fellow, Department of Plastic Surgery, Chang Gung Memorial Hospital, Chang Gung University and Medical College, Taiwan

Iain S Whitaker BA (Hons), MA Cantab, MB BChir, MRCS
Specialist Registrar in Burns and Plastic Surgery, Welsh Centre for Burns and Plastic Surgery, Morriston Hospital, Swansea, Wales

Nicholas Wilson-Jones MB BCh, MSc, MRCS (Ed), FRCS (Plast)
Consultant Paediatric Plastic Surgeon, Welsh Centre for Burns and Plastic Surgery, Morriston Hospital, Swansea, Wales

Editorial Assistant

Charles Stalnaker Brown BS
Plastic Surgery Research Fellow, University of Louisville School of Medicine, Louisville, Kentucky, USA

Preface

The final examination is one endpoint in the training pathway of the plastic surgeon - but there are others, and this important perspective must not be forgotten in the approach that any young surgeon in training has towards their education in the specialty. The questions in this book have been designed to test not only the factual knowledge base, but also an understanding of the key principles of plastic surgery. While the questions are based upon the various higher examination structures (Boards, EBOPRAS, FRCS, MCh), they are intended to be challenging and provide readers with a gauge of their abilities as well as an aid to study and revision. Some questions may not be in the syllabus of all jurisdictions for examination purposes, but the knowledge base required or gained in the process of reading this book is intended to enrich the learning experience of the reader and gives a firm base upon which further knowledge can be built.

Kayvan Shokrollahi BSc MB ChB MSc LLM MRCS (Eng) FRCS (Plast)
Specialist Registrar in Burns and Plastic Surgery

Iain S Whitaker BA (Hons) MA Cantab MB BChir MRCS
Specialist Registrar in Burns and Plastic Surgery

Hamish Laing BSc MBBS FRCS (Plast)
Consultant Plastic Surgeon
Communications Officer of the British Association of Plastic,
Reconstructive and Aesthetic Surgeons (BAPRAS)

About the editors

Kayvan Shokrollahi graduated from Bristol University with both a Bachelor of Science degree with first-class honours in Cellular and Molecular Pathology (1996) and a degree in Medicine (1999). He went on to graduate with both a Master of Science degree in Clinical Engineering and a Master of Laws degree with commendation. His basic training was undertaken in Bristol where he gained the Membership Diploma (MRCS) of The Royal College of Surgeons of England in 2002. He undertook parts of his training in various aspects of plastic surgery in a number of units in the UK including Oxford, Chester, Swansea, the Canniesburn unit in Glasgow, and also the Children's Hospital in Los Angeles, and has been awarded fellowships in Nottingham, UK, and Ottawa in Canada. He became a Hunterian Professor of The Royal College of Surgeons of England in 2007 and gained his specialist fellowship diploma in plastic surgery FRCS (Plast) in 2009. He has won prizes from the British Association of Plastic, Reconstructive and Aesthetic Surgeons, Bristol University and the Pathological Society of Great Britain. He is on the editorial board of a number of journals, including his role as Associate Editor at the *Annals of Plastic Surgery*, having published extensively in medical journals and books. He peer reviews for a number of plastic surgery journals including the *Journal of Plastic, Reconstructive and Aesthetic Surgery*. He has an interest in medical education, having been an Honorary Lecturer in presentation skills, is an advisor to the National Library for Health, and has developed courses for interview and viva voce training. He is also an accomplished pianist-composer with weekly radio performances of his original music on rotation on national classical radio stations in Europe such as Classic FM and Klassikradio under the pseudonym Shokolat.

Iain Whitaker read medicine at Trinity Hall College, University of Cambridge, where he also obtained the degrees of Bachelor and Master of Arts. Iain completed his subinternship in plastic surgery at Harvard Medical School, USA, followed by his surgical house officer post at Addenbrooke's Hospital in Cambridge. After serving as an anatomy demonstrator at the University of Cambridge, he completed his general surgery training in the Yorkshire School of Surgery, and subsequently became a Member of The Royal College of Surgeons. During his specialist training at the Welsh Centre for Burns and Plastic Surgery, he has spent time overseas in both clinical and research activities in Uppsala (Sweden), Louisville and Connecticut (USA). Iain has published over 100 peer-reviewed papers, several book chapters and books. He has won academic awards from Cambridge University, The Royal College of Surgeons, the British Association of Plastic, Reconstructive and Aesthetic Surgeons (BAPRAS) and commercial bodies. He is an Associate Editor for the *Annals of Plastic Surgery*, and is a peer reviewer for the *Journal of Plastic, Reconstructive and Aesthetic Surgery* (JPRAS), *Microsurgery* and *Burns*. He is involved in collaborative research with Uppsala, Louisville, Connecticut and Melbourne while completing his PhD thesis.

Hamish Laing graduated in medicine from London where he also obtained a first-class honours degree in Physiology and the University Prize. During his training he has held both clinical and research appointments at several of the United Kingdom's top centres including Mount Vernon Hospital, the RAFT Institute, The Great Ormond Street Hospital for Children and The Royal Marsden Hospital. He has published widely in the plastic surgery literature, including book chapters for international texts on hand surgery. Now a Consultant Plastic and Reconstructive Surgeon at the Welsh Centre for Burns and Plastic Surgery with a special interest in skin cancer and upper limb surgery, he is a national clinical lead for Sarcoma. In addition to his clinical commitments, Hamish is the Communications Officer of the British Association of Plastic, Reconstructive and Aesthetic Surgeons (BAPRAS), National Advisor for Plastic Surgery in Wales, a member of the Faculty for Healthcare Improvement and Associated Medical Director in his Trust.

Editorial Assistant

Charles Stalnaker Brown is a medical student and a research fellow in the Plastic Surgery Research laboratories at the University of Louisville. He graduated magna cum laude from the University of Louisville with a BS in Biology and his current research interests focus on composite tissue allotransplantation, facial reconstruction, bioengineering, and general plastic surgery. He is anticipating entering an integrated plastic surgery residency program in the near future.

Acknowledgements

We are grateful to the many international experts for their contributions to this text. Their efforts highlight the great importance of education and mentorship, and to them we owe a great debt.

We are indebted to Charles Stalnaker Brown who has worked on the project as Editorial Assistant.

We are very grateful to Mr William Norbury for proof reading the text with a knowledgeable critical eye.

It is with great sadness that we report the passing of one of our contributors, Professor Paolo Santoni-Rugiu (1928-2009), during the final stages of manuscript production. Along with Mr Philip Sykes, he produced an excellent section on the history of plastic surgery. His dedication to plastic surgery training was immense, and he will be sadly missed by his many colleagues and friends around the world.

We are especially grateful to Nikki Bramhill and her colleagues at tfm publishing for seeing the potential of this project, and guiding us through the publication process so smoothly.

Guidance notes

NOTES ON CONTENT

The international contributors to this manuscript have provided over half of the questions herein. The editors between them have written over 150 questions. The questions have all been edited for content and style to ensure an appropriate and matched level of difficulty, clarity and unambiguity. Each question is often an amalgam of the concerted efforts of many individuals.

APPROACH TO QUESTIONS AND ANSWERS

Almost every question has **ONE** correct answer from **FIVE** provided. This should be assumed unless stated otherwise. The occasional question is in a different format and, as with any examination, readers should ensure they read the question thoroughly to avoid mistakes.

Section 1 questions

Basic principles and basic science

1 Which one of the following is true regarding collagen?

A. Its derivation is debated: either from the Greek for 'strength' or the Latin for 'strand'.
B. Type 1 collagen is formed from three identical 'alpha' chains.
C. Type 3 collagen is formed from two different 'alpha' chains.
D. Every third amino acid in collagen is glycine, the others usually being proline and hydroxyproline.
E. Collagen is stabilized by polymerization.

2 With regards to anticoagulants in microsurgery:

A. Heparin and antithrombin III have similar mechanisms of action.
B. Unfractionated and fractionated heparins have different proportions of anti-Factor Xa and antithrombin activity.
C. Heparin-induced thrombocytopenia is a more frequent complication of unfractionated prophylactic heparin than of fractionated prophylactic heparin use.
D. The antiplatelet drug aspirin is contraindicated in patients younger than 16 years of age.
E. Dextran anticoagulation is pharmacologically reversible.

3 Which landmark publication related to free tissue transfer is correct?

A. The first successful thumb replantation was performed by Komatsu and Tamai in 1967.
B. The first clinical series of free tissue transfers was published by Nakayama in 1969.
C. Cobbett performed the first successful free great toe-to-hand transfer in humans in 1968.
D. McLean and Buncke performed the first free omentum flap in 1971.
E. None of the above is true.

4 Concerning composite tissue allotransplantation, which of the following is true?

A. Corticosteroids are used for both maintenance therapy and treatment of acute rejection episodes and act by inhibiting NF-κB activation and inflammatory cytokine production.
B. Antithymocyte globulin (ATG) is an induction agent which binds cell surface antigens, and depletes T cells.
C. Tacrolimus (FK 506) blocks the production of IL-2 and has been shown in recent studies to possibly speed up nerve regrowth.
D. Mycophenolate mofetil (MMF) prevents T-cell proliferation and differentiation.
E. All of the above.

5 In relation to free tissue transfer, which one is true?

A. The anterolateral thigh free flap, by definition, is based on the descending branch of the lateral circumflex femoral artery.
B. The superficial inferior epigastric artery pedicle is absent in approximately 5% of cases.
C. The skin paddle of the fibula osteoseptocutaneous free flap is an unreliable indicator of the blood supply to the fibula bone.

D.   Some surgeons are capable of performing microsurgery without the aid of a surgical microscope.
E.   None of the above is true.

6   According to Mathes and Nahai:

A.   The posterior interosseous artery flap is a Type C fasciocutaneous flap.
B.   The lateral arm flap is a Type C fasciocutaneous flap.
C.   The scapular flap is a Type C fasciocutaneous flap.
D.   The deltopectoral flap is a Type C fasciocutaneous flap.
E.   None of the above is true.

3

7   With regards to toe-to-hand transfer:

A.   The dominant blood supply to the great toe is the first plantar metatarsal artery in 25% of cases and the first dorsal metatarsal artery in 75% of cases.
B.   A metacarpal hand results when all its fingers have been amputated proximal to the proximal phalanx, with or without thumb involvement.
C.   Repair of the toe extensor tendon(s) in the hand should be performed after an accurate finger cascade has been achieved by flexor tendon repair(s).
D.   When reconstructing a Type IIC metacarpal hand by toe-to-hand transplantations, finger reconstruction should usually precede thumb reconstruction.
E.   Nicoladoni was the first to report pedicled great toe-to-hand transfer.

8   Regarding free tissue transfer:

A.   According to Koshima, supramicrosurgery (or supermicrosurgery) is defined as microvascular dissection and anastomosis of vessels measuring less than 0.5mm.
B.   In 1960, Jacobson and Suarez reported successful experimental microvascular anastomoses as small as 0.9mm in diameter.

C. The first successful free tissue transfer in humans was performed in America.
D. Taylor is credited with the first description of the free fibula osteocutaneous flap.
E. None of the above is true.

9 The dominant type of collagen in tendon is:

A. Type I.
B. Type II.
C. Type V.
D. Type IV.
E. Type III.

10 The dorsal artery of the penis is immediately deep to which anatomical layer?

A. Skin.
B. Tunica albuginea.
C. Buck fascia.
D. Dartos fascia.
E. Tunica vaginalis.

11 Which of these conditions is a disorder of collagen?

A. Marfan's syndrome.
B. Cutis laxa.
C. Progeria.
D. Osteogenesis imperfecta.
E. Pallister-Hall syndrome.

12 Body mass index is calculated:

A. By a ratio of soft tissue mass to bone mass.
B. By multiplying height (in metres) by weight (in kilograms).
C. By dividing body weight (in kilograms) by a bone density factor.
D. By dividing twice the body weight (in kilograms) by half the height in metres.
E. By dividing body weight in kilograms by the square of body height in metres.

13 In order to practice evidence-based plastic surgery, a knowledge of statistical concepts is important. The following statements are true except:

A. Regression analysis is used to find how one set of data relates to another.
B. Correlation measures the strength of the association between variables.
C. The Chi-square test is a measure of the difference between actual and expected frequencies.
D. The mode is the point which has half the values above and half the values below.
E. The P value gives the probability of any observed difference having happened by chance.

14 Tissue expansion:

A. May be used in conjunction with component separation to allow primary closure of abdominal defects involving 25% or less of the abdominal surface area.
B. In the extremities has been associated with higher levels of complications.
C. Is useful in the acute management of lower limb soft tissue trauma.
D. Is associated with more complications in upper extremities than lower extremities.
E. Tap water is reasonable to use for inflation.

15 The flexor hallucis muscle has the following pattern of blood supply according to Mathes and Nahai:

A. I.
B. II.
C. III.
D. IV.
E. V.

16 A Z-plasty is an example of:

A. An advancement flap.
B. A delayed flap.
C. An island pedicle flap.
D. A rotation flap.
E. A transposition flap.

17 Compared to the free deep inferior epigastric artery perforator (DIEP) flap, the free transverse rectus abdominis myocutaneous (TRAM) flap has:

A. Less donor site morbidity.
B. More problems with venous drainage of the flap.
C. A better survival of zone IV.
D. Fewer problems with infection.
E. Longer admission periods.

18 The primary source of blood to the lower half of the central abdominal skin is the:

A. Superficial inferior epigastric artery.
B. Deep inferior epigastric artery.
C. Superior epigastric artery.
D. Superficial circumflex iliac artery.
E. Intercostal and segmental arteries.

19 Thinning of a paramedian forehead flap for nasal reconstruction is:

A. Never safe.
B. Only feasible at the distal 1cm of the flap.
C. Safest if performed at an intermediate stage.
D. Best performed by thinning the forehead skin by tissue expansion.
E. In general not necessary to achieve a good result.

20 In order to practice evidence-based plastic surgery, a knowledge of statistical concepts is important. The following statements are true except:

A. The Mann-Whitney U test is a non-parametric test.
B. The Kruskal-Wallis test is a non-parametric test.
C. A meta-analysis is a method of combining results from a number of independent studies to give an overall estimate of effect.
D. Non-parametric tests are dependent on the distribution of the data.
E. The normal distribution of data is symmetrical, forming a characteristic bell-shaped curve.

21 The names of Salmon, Manchot, Taylor, Morain, and Tempest are all associated with our knowledge of which of the following?

A. Microsurgery.
B. Breast reconstruction.
C. Blood supply to skin.
D. Nerve supply to skin.
E. Free flap reconstruction.

22 To prevent microvascular anastomosis occlusion in a standard microsurgical case you should:

A.   Keep the operating theatre temperature high.
B.   Make sure both vessels are of the same calibre.
C.   Make sure there is no intimal damage in either vessel.
D.   Inject a bolus of heparin before putting the clamp on the vessel.
E.   Never release the vein before starting the arterial anastomosis.

23 Which of the following statements is false?

A.   Polyglactic acid (Vicryl®) is a synthetic polyfilament suture which loses its tensile strength after 4-5 weeks and is said to be absorbed at 3 months.
B.   Polydioxanone (PDS®) is a synthetic monofilament suture which loses its tensile strength after 3 weeks and is absorbed at 2 months.
C.   Polypropylene (Prolene®), a polymer of propylene, is a monofilament, non-absorbable suture which can be used to repair fascia, tendon, muscle and vessels.
D.   'Catgut' sutures are derived from sheep intestine, lose their tensile strength after 7-10 days, and are absorbed at 2 months.
E.   All of the above.

24 Which statement is false?

A.   The parascapular flap is vascularised by the transverse branch of the circumflex scapular vessels.
B.   The anterolateral thigh flap is normally vascularised by the descending branch of the lateral circumflex femoral vessels.
C.   The skin island of the osteocutaneous fibula free flap is generally circulated by septocutaneous branches from the peroneal vessels running off posterior of the fibula.
D.   The venous outflow of the radial forearm flap can be based on either the concomitant veins of the radial artery or on the cephalic vein or on both.
E.   The scapular angle is circulated through the angular branch which comes from the thoracodorsal vessels.

25 When a free flap is failing due to venous or arterial thrombosis:

A.   Do not re-explore because the salvage rate is low.
B.   It is reasonable to re-explore the next day.
C.   The use of streptokinase is the procedure of choice.
D.   Administer IV heparin and wait.
E.   It is necessary to attempt removal of the entire propagated clot.

26 Mathes and Nahai described muscle flaps. Within this same classification, they also described a number of non-muscle flaps. Which of these flaps is correctly attributed?

A.   Fibula flap - Type V.
B.   Omental flap - Type III.
C.   Jejunum flap - Type I.
D.   All of the above.
E.   None of the above.

27 The following landmark paper or author is not appropriately attributed:

A.   Huger (1976) - zones of abdominal wall blood supply.
B.   Cuthbertson (1942, *Lancet*) - the hypermetabolic response to injury (rodent study).
C.   Boca (1906) - radical neck dissection.
D.   Winter (1962, *Nature*) - moist wounds heal better.
E.   Penn (1955) - ideal breast measurements.

28 The following is the appropriate treatment postoperatively for patients with split skin grafts to the lower limb:

A. Ten days of bed rest.
B. Next day wound check and discharge.
C. Use of a warming blanket, but only in patients over 50 years of age.
D. Opioid analgesia.
E. None of the above.

29 Name the flap which is not a part of the subscapular vascular axis:

A. Serratus anterior flap.
B. Latissimus dorsi flap.
C. Intercostal artery perforator flap (ICAP).
D. Parascapular flap.
E. Thoracodorsal perforator (TAP) flap.

30 Following tissue expansion:

A. The thickness of the dermis increases as the skin is expanded.
B. The mitotic rate of skin stays static during expansion.
C. The thickness of the epidermis tends to increase.
D. The stratum lucidum thickens by at least 75%.
E. Hair density is not reduced in expanded skin.

31 Which one of the following is true?

A. The anterior tibial artery can be found between extensor hallucis longus and extensor digitorum longus in the proximal third of the leg.
B. The direct source artery for the anterolateral thigh flap is the femoral artery.
C. The surface landmark for the posterior tibial artery is a line drawn from the medial border of the patella to the medial malleolus.

D. A hemi-soleus muscle flap can be raised on the same vascular axis as the fibula flap.
E. The first dorsal metatarsal artery usually arises from the posterior tibial artery.

32 For a 4cm x 4cm defect on the weight-bearing surface of the heel, the ideal reconstruction would be:

A. Innervated radial forearm free flap.
B. Free gracilis and skin graft.
C. Reverse sural artery flap.
D. Free or pedicled dorsalis pedis flap.
E. Sensate pedicled medial plantar island flap.

33 Large fasciocutaneous flaps include all except:

A. Groin flap.
B. Thoracodorsal artery perforator flap.
C. Anterolateral thigh flap.
D. First dorsal metacarpal artery flap.
E. Deltopectoral flap.

34 Which one of the following organs or tissues is considered to be the most immunogenic following allograft transplantation?

A. Kidney.
B. Heart.
C. Skin.
D. Pancreas.
E. All have the same immunogenicity.

35 Whose research work challenged the 'length vs breadth' principle for flap dimensions popularised by Gillies?

A. Taylor.
B. O'Brien.
C. Milton.
D. Salmon.
E. Blair.

36 Which statement is true?

A. The gracilis muscle is a poor choice for perineal reconstruction due to its small width.
B. The adductor artery usually arises from the profunda femoris artery but it may also arise from the medial circumflex artery.
C. A gracilis flap is not a viable option for breast reconstruction.
D. The obturator nerve supplies the motor innervation to the gracilis muscle.
E. The muscle tendons found at the medial aspect of the knee from superficial to deep are encountered in the following order: gracilis, sartorius, semimembranosus.

37 Who served as Medical Officer with Garibaldi and has a name associated with the full thickness skin graft?

A. Moretti.
B. Wolfe.
C. Santoni.
D. Ollier.
E. Baronio.

38 Interleukin-1 (IL-1) is released from:

A. Platelets.
B. Collagen.
C. Neutrophils.
D. Fibroblasts.
E. Endothelium.

39 Concerning foetal wound healing:

A. Scarring is similar to adults.
B. There are higher concentrations of Type III collagen.
C. There are lower concentrations of hyaluronic acid.
D. There are higher concentrations of Type IV collagen.
E. Concentrations of hyaluronic acid are the same.

40 The following best describes the sequence of sensory recovery in a healing skin graft:

A. Temperature, pain, light touch.
B. Pain, temperature, light touch.
C. Pain, light touch, temperature.
D. Light touch, pain, temperature.
E. Temperature, light touch, pain.

41 Regarding free tissue transfer:

A. Primary then secondary ischaemia are mandatory events for free tissue transfer to proceed.
B. The no-reflow phenomenon is peculiar to free tissue transfer.
C. A pseudo-intima forms within a successful microvascular anastomosis after approximately 10 days.
D. The presence of subendothelial damage will cause anastomotic thrombosis and failure.
E. None of the above is true.

42 Following split thickness skin grafting:

A. The mitotic activity is static.
B. The nuclei and cytoplasm decrease in size.
C. The epithelium increases in thickness during the first 3 weeks.
D. Enzymic activity increases in the first 3 days.
E. The fibrocyte population increases in the first 3 days post-graft.

43 After the age of 35:

A. The dermis gradually thickens.
B. Skin elasticity increases.
C. Sebaceous gland content increases
D. The dermis gradually thins.
E. There is no loss of sebaceous gland content.

44 At the site of a microvascular anastomosis the following events occur in the correct order:

A. Pseudo-intima, platelet aggregation, fibrin formation, endothelium.
B. Fibrin formation, platelet aggregation, endothelium, pseudo-intima.
C. Platelet aggregation, fibrin formation, pseudo-intima, endothelium.
D. Fibrin formation, platelet aggregation, pseudo-intima, endothelium.
E. None of the above.

45 The lateral arm free flap is based on:

A. The posterior radial collateral artery.
B. The anterior radial collateral artery.
C. The posterior ulnar collateral artery.
D. The anterior ulnar collateral artery.
E. The lateral circumflex humeral artery.

46 According to the Mathes and Nahai classification, sartorius is:

A.   A Type I muscle flap.
B.   A Type II muscle flap.
C.   A Type III muscle flap.
D.   A Type IV muscle flap.
E.   A Type V muscle flap.

47 Concerning anticoagulation:

A.   Heparin decreases the efficacy of antithrombin III.
B.   Dextran is a polysaccharide.
C.   The action of aspirin is reversible at the molecular level.
D.   The intrinsic and extrinsic pathways converge at Factor 9.
E.   Dextran imparts a positive charge to platelets.

48 The groin flap is usually based on:

A.   The deep circumflex iliac artery.
B.   The lateral circumflex iliac artery.
C.   The superficial inferior epigastric artery.
D.   The superficial circumflex femoral artery.
E.   The superficial circumflex iliac artery.

49 Papaverine:

A.   Is an opium alkaloid.
B.   Is a vasoconstrictor.
C.   Inhibits phosphodiesterase and reduces cAMP levels.
D.   Is a local anaesthetic.
E.   May not be applied directly to blood vessels.

50 The following key paper is not appropriately attributed:

A.   Allen (1994, *Ann Plast Surg*) - the first description of the DIEP flap.
B.   Argenta and Morykwas (1997, *Ann Plast Surg*) - the description of vacuum-assisted wound closure.
C.   Matarasso (1995, *Ann Plast Surg*) - classification related to abdominoplasty.
D.   Cordeiro (2002, *Plast Reconstr Surg*) - classification and algorithm for acquired vaginal defects.
E.   Rohrich (2003, *Ann Plast Surg*) - classification of gynaecomastia in relation to suction-assisted lipectomy.

51 Concerning leech therapy used to salvage venously congested tissues, which of the following is false?

A.   Complications include postoperative infection with *Aeromonas spp.*
B.   Augmentin® is the most effective prophylactic antibiotic.
C.   The gastro-intestinal microbiota differs between *Hirudo* spp.
D.   *Hirudo medicinalis* was FDA approved as a medical device in 2004.
E.   Recent microbiological studies have shown that *Aeromonas* is sensitive to fluoroquinolones.

52 When vein grafts are used to bridge intra-arterial defects:

A.   The vein wall thins due to the increased luminal pressure.
B.   Graft length decreases by 25-30% long term.
C.   The graft stretches by 20-30%
D.   The vein wall thickens significantly.
E.   There is no ingrowth of smooth muscle cells.

53 The rupture rate of silicone breast implants is approximately:

A. 5% at 5 years.
B. 5% at 10 years.
C. 50% at 5 years.
D. 50% at 12 years.
E. 15% at 15 years.

54 The following statements concerning hyaluronic acid are true except:

A. It is found in the vitreous humour of the eye.
B. It is a major constituent of Perlane®.
C. It is a major constituent of Radiesse®.
D. It is a glycosaminoglycan.
E. It is not available as an oral preparation.

55 The four zones within the capsule surrounding an expander were described by:

A. Radovan.
B. Neumann.
C. Paysk.
D. Brand.
E. Nalebuff.

56 The following statement is incorrect regarding local anaesthetic administration:

A. The maximum dose for lignocaine infiltration is 4mg/kg.
B. The maximum dose for lignocaine + adrenaline (epinephrine) infiltration is 7mg/kg.
C. Warming the solution may reduce the pain of administration.

D.   Rate of subcutaneous injection rarely influences the perception of pain by the patient.

E.   Adding hyaluronidase is a useful technique for the harvesting of split thickness skin grafts.

57 Requirements for successful and effective microsurgical training:

A.   Good hand-eye co-ordination.
B.   Patience of candidates and tutors.
C.   Appropriate educational centres and training programs.
D.   Individualised advanced training.
E.   All of the above is true.

58 After serious ischaemia of tissues in the microcirculation the 'no-reflow' phenomenon can appear, that consists of several events and factors except for:

A.   Microvascular spasm.
B.   Interstitial oedema.
C.   Microthrombi.
D.   Myoglobinuria.
E.   Swollen myocytes compressing vessel.

Section 1 answers

Basic principles and basic science

Answers

19

1 D.

Every third amino acid in collagen is glycine, the others usually being proline and hydroxyproline. Collagen is derived from the Greek *kolla* (glue) and *gennao* (to produce) because when boiled, collagen forms glue. The fibrillar collagens, Type 1 and 3, are the most abundant types in skin. Type 1 is comprised of polypeptide chains which are arranged in a triple helix. Two of the chains making up Type 1 collagen are identical (alpha-1 chain), while the third chain is distinct (alpha-2 chain). Every third amino acid in the collagen molecule is glycine, resulting in the pattern Gly-X-Y with the X and Y positions occupied by proline and hydroxyproline. Stability is due to disulphide bonds and also cross-links formed as a result of de-amination of lysyl and hydroxylysyl residues. Type 3 collagen is expressed in greater quantities in scar and healing tissue, and Type 4 collagen is found in the basement membrane.

2 B.

Unfractionated and fractionated heparins have different proportions of anti-Factor Xa and antithrombin activity. Heparin exerts its anticoagulant activity principally by binding antithrombin III. This causes increased exposure of the antithrombin III active site that, in turn, inactivates the coagulation enzymes, Factor IIa, IXa and Xa. Fractionated heparins also bind antithrombin III but have greater anti-Factor Xa activity rather than greater antithrombin activity. The frequency of heparin-induced thrombocytopenia varies greatly depending on, amongst other factors, the type of heparin administered and the patient population receiving it. In a large clinical trial, serologically-confirmed heparin-induced thrombocytopenia was approximately 1% at 7 days and 3% at 14 days in patients receiving prophylactic unfractionated heparin and 0% in patients receiving prophylactic fractionated heparin. Aspirin is contraindicated in patients under the age of 16 years when used other than as an antiplatelet agent (due to the risk of Reye's syndrome).

References

1.   Warkentin TE, Levine MN, Hirsh J, Horsewood P, Roberts RS, Gent M, Kelton JG. Heparin-induced thrombocytopenia in patients treated with low-molecular-weight heparin or unfractionated heparin. *N Engl J Med* 1995; 332: 1330.

3   C.

Cobbett performed the first successful free great toe-to-hand transfer in humans in 1968. Komatsu and Tamai performed the first known successful thumb replantation in 1965 and published their accomplishment in 1968. Nakayama published the first clinical series of free tissue transfers in 1964 (16 of 21 were successful; all were performed without a surgical microscope). Although it has been published that toe-to-hand free tissue transfer in humans was first performed in China in 1967, this was of the second toe; Cobbett was the first to perform free great toe-to-hand transfer in humans. McLean and Buncke performed the first free omentum flap in 1969 for scalp reconstruction and published their achievement in 1972.

4   E.

All of the above. The ultimate goal, and thus the focus of transplant immunology research, is to effectively suppress rejection while minimising toxic side effects. In clinical practice this is achieved through a balance of multiple drugs that interfere with the immune response at various sites by blocking the formation, stimulation, proliferation, and differentiation of lymphocytes. These drugs are administered immediately after transplanting the organ or tissues (induction therapy) and regularly thereafter 'for life' (maintenance therapy) and in response to rejection episodes (treatment or rescue therapy). The above drugs are often used following composite tissue allotransplantation.

References

1.   Whitaker IS, Duggan EM, Alloway RR, Brown CS, McGuire S, Woodle ES, Hsiao EC, Maldonado C, Banis JC, Jr., Barker JH. Composite tissue allotransplantation: a review of relevant immunological issues for plastic surgeons. *J Plast Reconstr Aesthet Surg* 2008; 61(5): 481-92.

5   E.

None of the above is true. The skin of the anterolateral thigh can be based on any appropriate underlying pedicle, which may or may not arise from the descending branch of the lateral circumflex femoral artery. The superficial inferior epigastric artery was absent in 35% of cadaveric dissections and in 40% of patients in a clinical study. Although the skin paddle of the fibula osteoseptocutaneous free flap was widely believed to be unreliable during the 1970s and 1980s, this has been refuted by several clinical studies from different centres. Microsurgery is, by definition, performed with the aid of a surgical microscope.

References

1.   Semple JL. Retrograde microvascular augmentation (turbocharging) of a single-pedicle TRAM flap through a deep inferior epigastric arterial and venous loop. *Plast Reconstr Surg* 1994; 93(1): 109-17.

2.   Taylor GI, Caddy CM, Watterson Paul A, Crock JG. The venous territories (venosomes) of the human body: experimental study and clinical implications. *Plast Reconstr Surg* 1990; 86(2): 185-213.

3.   Wei FC, Chen HC, Chuang CC, Noordhoff MS. Fibular osteoseptocutaneous flap: anatomic study and clinical application. *Plast Reconstr Surg* 1986; 78: 191.

4.   Hidalgo DA. Fibula free flap: a new method of mandible reconstruction. *Plast Reconstr Surg* 1989; 84: 71.

6   D.

The deltopectoral flap is a Type C fasciocutaneous flap. The others are Type B fasciocutaneous flaps. Type A flaps are supplied by direct cutaneous vessels, Type B are septocutaneous and Type C are musculocutaneous. Cormack and Lamberty also classified fasciocutaneous flaps. Type A flaps are supplied by un-named vessels entering at the base of the flap, Type B flaps have an axial vessel, and Type C have segmental perforators from a deeper source vessel.

7 D.

When reconstructing a Type IIC metacarpal hand by toe-to-hand transplantations, finger reconstruction should usually precede thumb reconstruction. In approximately 10% of cases, the first dorsal and plantar metatarsal arteries are co-dominant. A metacarpal hand results when all fingers have been amputated proximal to the middle of the proximal phalanx, with (Type II) or without (Type I) thumb involvement. Types I and II metacarpal hands are subdivided further according to the levels of finger and thumb amputations, respectively. Type IIC metacarpal hands additionally have inadequate thenar muscular function; finger reconstruction by toe transfer(s) should therefore precede thumb reconstruction to ensure restoration of accurate digital prehension. The toe extensor tendon repairs in the hand during toe-to-hand transfer should be performed under tension and before flexor tendon repair in order to reduce the risk of neo-digit clawing thereafter. Nicoladoni reported pedicled second toe-to-hand transfer.

8 C.

The first successful free tissue transfer in humans was performed in America. The first successful free tissue transfer in humans was performed without a surgical microscope by Seidenberg *et al* in 1957 in Montefiore Hospital, New York City, and reported 2 years later. Supermicrosurgery is defined as microvascular dissection and anastomosis of small-calibre vessels measuring 0.5 to 0.8mm in diameter. Jacobson and Suarez reported successful microvascular anastomoses in vessels down to 1.4mm in diameter. Taylor is credited with the first description of the free fibula osseous flap without a skin paddle, and he also described the deep circumflex iliac artery (DCIA) flap.

References

1.   Koshima I. Superficial circumflex iliac artery perforator flap. In: *Perforator flaps: anatomy, technique, & clinical applications.* Blondeel PN, Morris SF, Hallock GG, Neligan PC, Eds. St. Louis, USA: Quality Medical Publishing, 2006: 977.

2.   Seidenberg B, Rosenak SS, Hurwitt ES, Som ML. Immediate reconstruction of the cervical esophagus by a revascularized isolated jejunal segment. *Ann Surg* 1959; 149(2): 162-71.

9   A.

Type I.

10   C.

Buck fascia. Anatomical layers of the dorsal penile shaft, from external inwards, are: skin, dartos fascia, Buck (deep) fascia and tunica albuginea. The superficial arterial plexus lies within dartos fascia and supplies the skin and prepuce but the dorsal artery of the penis lies beneath Buck (deep) fascia. The tunica vaginalis is in the scrotum.

11   D.

Osteogenesis imperfecta. Osteogenesis imperfecta is a disorder of Type 1 collagen. Marfan's syndrome is a disorder of fibrillin (a component of microfibrils in elastic tissue). Cutis laxa is a disorder of elastin and Progeria is a disorder of lamin A (a component of nuclear lamina). Pallister-Hall is a rare syndrome associated with polydactyly.

12   E.

By dividing body weight in kilograms by the square of body height in metres.

13   D.

The mode is the point which has half the values above and half the values below. This statement is incorrect; the mode is NOT the point which has half the values above and half the values below. This defines the median. The mode is the single value that occurs most frequently.

14 B.

In the extremities has been associated with higher levels of complications. Adequate reconstruction is usually achieved despite these complications when the technique is used.

15 D.

IV. The supply is via multiple segmental vessels. Many of the flexor and extensor muscles of the lower limb have this pattern, so it is actually easy to remember: flexor digitorum, flexor hallucis, extensor digitorum, extensor hallucis and tibialis anterior all have Type IV supply.

16 E.

A transposition flap. Z-plasty is an example of a transposition flap.

17 E.

Longer admission periods. A longer admission period is the feature with most robust evidence. Some would argue there is less donor site morbidity but strong evidence for this is lacking. There is no difference in the incidence of abdominal hernias between the two techniques.

18 B.

Deep inferior epigastric artery. This pattern of blood supply was extensively described by Huger.

19 c.

Safest if performed at an intermediate stage. Thinning of the paramedian forehead flap can be performed at the initial stage; however, it can result in compromised flap circulation. Aggressive subdermal thinning is safest at an intermediate stage after 2-3 weeks when the circulation of the flap has been increased by the delay phenomenon.

20 d.

Non-parametric tests are dependent on the distribution of the data. This statement is incorrect; non-parametric tests are actually independent of the distribution of the data.

21 c.

Blood supply to skin. Carl Manchot wrote about the blood supply of the skin in 1889 and Michel-Marie Salmon used radio opaque preservatives to investigate the arteries of the skin in 1936. Manchot's work was reviewed by Morain in 1985 and Salmon's was translated and edited by Taylor and Tempest in 1988.

22 c.

Make sure there is no intimal damage in either vessel. The only real issue is to have good flow with undamaged intima and no debris inside the vessel or at the anastomotic site in a standard case with no other associated blood clotting or trauma issues.

23 b.

Polydioxanone (PDS®) is a synthetic monofilament suture which loses its tensile strength after 3 weeks and is absorbed at 2 months. PDS sutures maintain tensile strength for up to 8 weeks, and take up to 6 months to absorb.

24 A.

The parascapular flap is vascularised by the transverse branch of the circumflex scapular vessels. A is false; the parascapular flap is supplied by the descending branch; the scapula flap is supplied by the transverse branch.

25 E.

It is necessary to attempt removal of the entire propagated clot.

26 D.

All of the above. The fibula has a dominant supply from the peroneal artery with additional multiple segmental vessels along its length. Classic Type V muscle flaps include latissimus dorsi and pectoralis major. The omentum has a dual blood supply from the left and right gastro-epiploic artery. Classic Type III muscle flaps include gluteus maximus and rectus abdominis. The jejunum is supplied by the superior mesenteric artery. Classic Type I muscle flaps include gastrocnemius and tensor fascia lata. Taylor classified flaps according to their nerve supply, and Mathes and Nahai, as well as Cormack and Lamberty, classified fasciocutaneous flaps.

27 C.

Boca (1906) - radical neck dissection. This is incorrect; Crile first described the radical neck dissection, and Boca the functional neck dissection. Huger described the abdominal wall vascularity, which in simple terms comprises inferior, central and lateral zones. Winter showed that moist wounds heal better in a classic article in *Nature*, although this has been challenged. Penn objectively scrutinised the breast aesthetic.

28 E.

None of the above. Early discharge is preferred. Many surgeons have different postoperative regimes for such patients. However, 10 days of bed rest has not been shown to improve graft take rates [1]. This prospective randomised controlled trial was conducted to compare the time to complete healing of patients mobilised early (the first postoperative day) against those who mobilised late (the tenth postoperative day). There was no difference in time to complete healing. Other problems with a bedrest strategy includes the increased risk to patients of deep venous thrombosis and pulmonary embolism - or instigation of prophylactic interventions such as heparin, as well as the risk of hospital-acquired infections with organisms such as MRSA. The actual and manpower costs are not justifiable. There is no benefit in checking a wound on the next postoperative day after grafting. Some advocate early dressing changes at 48 hours in case a haematoma is present which can be evacuated while the graft remains viable. Analgesia is usually required, in particular for the donor site, but opioids should not be required.

References
1.   Wood SH, Lees VC. A prospective investigation of the healing of grafted pretibial wounds with early and late mobilisation. *Br J Plast Surg* 1994; 47(2): 127-31.

29 C.

Intercostal artery perforator flap (ICAP). The subscapular artery divides into the circumflex scapula (parascapular) and the thoracodorsal arteries (latissimus dorsi and TAP flaps), which gives the serratus branch.

30 C.

The thickness of the epidermis tends to increase. The dermis and fat often thin.

31 D.

A hemi-soleus muscle flap can be raised on the same vascular axis as the fibula flap. The fibula flap is based on the peroneal artery, which gives a large branch to the lateral soleus just after dividing at the tibioperoneal trunk; this vessel is the major blood supply to the hemi-soleus but the skin perforators to the fibula can also provide an additional pedicle. The surface marking of the anterior tibial artery is a line between the anterior border of the head of the fibula to a midpoint between the two malleoli and the vessels can be exposed anywhere along this line. In the proximal third, the vascular bundle lies between tibialis anterior and extensor digitorum longus. Lower down, it lies between tibialis anterior and extensor hallucis longus. The surface marking for the posterior tibial artery is a line between the medial condyle of the tibia to a point 1cm posterior to the medial malleolus. The first dorsal metatarsal artery arises from the dorsalis pedis /anterior tibial artery.

32 E.

Sensate pedicled medial plantar island flap. Heel reconstruction needs to be resistant to stress and shear forces. The sensate, hairless, glabrous skin of the sole of the foot provides the ideal reconstruction for the weight bearing heel but its disadvantage is the skin graft on the sole of the foot. Muscle flaps require skin grafts and these are usually unstable and mostly insensate.

33 D.

First dorsal metacarpal artery flap. The first dorsal metacarpal artery flap is not large.

34 C.

Skin. Skin has long been regarded as a major barrier in composite tissue transplantation due to its high antigenicity. This strong immunogenicity is believed to be due to the presence of antigen presenting cells

(Langerhans cells), whose function is to present foreign antigens to the body's immune system.

35 C.

Milton. Milton did much of his work in Oxford and his famous paper on flaps on the flank of the pig was published in the *Brtish Journal of Plastic Surgery* in 1970.

36 D.

The obturator nerve supplies the motor innervation to the gracilis muscle. The nerve supply to the gracilis flap is the obturator nerve. The dominant vascular supply is the medial circumflex femoral artery and vein. At the medial knee, sartorius is superficial to gracilis and semitendinosus is deep. The gracilis musculocutaneous flap for breast reconstruction is well described, and gracilis is a workhorse flap in perineal reconstruction.

37 B.

Wolfe. Born in Breslau in 1824, he studied medicine in Glasgow and qualified in 1856. He worked as surgeon to Garibaldi's 'le Mille' in the Sicilian campaign in 1859 before returning to Scotland where he became an ophthalmic surgeon. He spent 8 years working in Melbourne from 1893, but returned to Glasgow and died in Scotland in 1904. He used full thickness skin grafts to avoid contracture when used on eyelids.

38 C.

Neutrophils.

39 B.

There are higher concentrations of Type III collagen. Furthermore, the inflammatory phase is absent or significantly attenuated in foetal healing.

40 C.

Pain, light touch, temperature.

41 E.

None of the above is true. Primary flap ischaemia is a mandatory event of free tissue transfer. Secondary (or tertiary, quaternary and so on) flap ischaemia occurs when the flap experiences another episode of ischaemia following revascularisation. A pseudo-intima usually lines the anastomosis by postoperative day five. The presence of subendothelial damage does not necessarily cause anastomotic thrombosis (and/or failure) but does influence the method by which the anastomosis heals. Therefore, none of the statements (A, B, C or D) are true.

42 C.

The epithelium increases in thickness during the first 3 weeks.

43 D.

The dermis gradually thins.

44 C.

Platelet aggregation, fibrin formation, pseudo-intima, endothelium. The events necessarily occur in the order shown in C. Platelet aggregation is required for fibrin formation which enables the formation of a pseudo-intima and endothelialisation.

45 A.

The posterior radial collateral artery.

46 D.

A Type IV muscle flap. The supply is segmental, and this is of relevance when using this flap such as for coverage of the femoral vessels during groin lymphadenectomy with a 'sartorius switch'. Some have suggested the proximal part of this flap is not viable during the switch procedure which simply scars and fibroses.

47 B.

31

Dextran is a polysaccharide. Heparin activates antithrombin III. The intrinsic and extrinsic coagulation pathways converge at Factor X. The antithrombotic effect of dextran is mediated through its binding of erythrocytes, platelets, and vascular endothelium, increasing their electronegativity and thus reducing erythrocyte aggregation and platelet adhesiveness. Dextrans also reduce Factor VIII-Ag von Willebrand Factor, thereby decreasing platelet function. Low-dose, long-term aspirin use irreversibly blocks the formation of thromboxane A2 in platelets, producing an inhibitory effect on platelet aggregation. Aspirin inhibits collagen-induced platelet aggregation and ADP-induced platelet aggregation, as well as blocking the release of ADP from platelets. ADP is known to be a potent platelet-aggregating substance. Aspirin acts on cyclo-oxygenase by causing irreversible acetylation of the enzyme, and therefore the effect is irreversible for the life of that platelet (7-10 days). Other non-steroidal anti-inflammatory analgesics have a reversible action on that enzyme, and hence only act until the drug is cleared from the circulation.

48 E.

The superficial circumflex iliac artery. However, Taylor's work argued for the advantages of raising the free groin flap based on the deep vessel [1, 2].

References
1.   Taylor GI, Townsend P, Corlett R. Superiority of the deep circumflex iliac vessels as the supply for free groin flaps. *Plast Reconstr Surg* 1979; 64(5): 595-604.

2.   Taylor GI, Townsend P, Corlett R. Superiority of the deep circumflex iliac vessels as the supply for free groin flaps. clinical work. *Plast Reconstr Surg* 1979; 64(6): 745-59.

3.   McGregor IA, Jackson IT. The groin flap. *Br J Plast Surg* 1972; 25(1): 3-16

4.   Smith PJ, Foley B, McGregor IA, Jackson IT. The anatomical basis of the groin flap. *Plast Reconstr Surg* 1972; 49(1): 41-7.

49 A.

Is an opium alkaloid. It is extracted from poppies but differs in both structure and pharmacological action from the other opiates. It acts through increasing cAMP levels via inhibition of phosphodiesterase leading to smooth muscle relaxation and vasodilation.

50 E.

Rohrich (2003, Ann Plast Surg) - classification of gynaecomastia in relation to suction-assisted lipectomy. This is incorrect; Rohrich published his classification of gynaecomastia in *Plastic Reconstructive Surgery* in relation to ultrasound-assisted lipectomy. The other papers are correctly attributed and all these papers would be a valuable addition to the reading list of readers.

51 B.

Augmentin® is the most effective prophylactic antibiotic. B is false. *Aeromonas* is a gram negative bacillus which is a well reported cause of infection following leech therapy. *Aeromonas spp.* strains resistant to Augmentin have been reported in several papers in the literature whereas fluoroquinolones seem to be consistently active. Recent microbiological studies have shown that the gastro-intestinal microbiota differs amongst the European medicinal leeches (*Hirudo verbana, orientalis* and *medicinalis*). Bacteria isolated from the leech include *Aeromonas veronii, rikenella* and *Morganella morganii.*

References

1.   Whitaker IS, Kamya C, Azzopardi EA, Graf J, Kon M, Lineaweaver WC. Preventing infective complications following leech therapy: is practice keeping pace with current research? *Microsurgery* 2009; Apr 27. [Epub ahead of print].

52 D.

The vein wall thickens significantly.

53 D.

50% at 12 years. This is the 'traditional' rate quoted [1]. However, many of these were older generation implants. More recent papers/data suggest a number closer to 10% at 10 years. Readers are recommended to re-appraise the future literature, and hence the validity of this answer.

References

1.   Robinson OG Jr, Bradley EL, Wilson DS. Analysis of explanted silicone implants: a report of 300 patients. *Ann Plast Surg* 1995; 34(1): 1-6.

54 C.

It is a major constituent of Radiesse®. C is false. Hyaluronan, also called hyaluronic acid or hyaluronate, is a non-sulfated glycosaminoglycan found in many tissues of the body, such as skin, cartilage, and the vitreous humour. Perlane® contains a much higher concentratation of hyaluronic acid than Restylane®. Radiesse comprises calcium hydroxyapatite particles. Hyaluronic acid can be found as oral preparations in health food shops and marketed commonly for arthritic ailments.

55 C.

Paysk. Tissue expansion was popularised by Neumann (1957) and Radovan (1975), and Austed undertook important work on histological changes in 1982.

56 D.

Rate of subcutaneous injection rarely influences the perception of pain by the patient. This statement is incorrect; increasing the rate of subcutaneous injection increases the pain. Warming and alkalinising the anaesthetic with bicarbonate also reduces the pain of infiltration. Although the 'safe' dose of lidocaine for direct infiltration is 4 or 7mg/kg with or without adrenaline (epinephrine), respectively, it can safely be used in much higher concentrations such as during tumescent infiltration for liposuction.

57 E.

All of the above is true. Effective microsurgical education is based on training centres with appropriate education programs, infrastructure and equipment. The individualised programs are more effective and require good hand-eye co-ordination, good manual skills and patience both of the participant and tutor.

References

1.   Furka I, Brath E, Nemeth N, Miko I. Learning microsurgical suturing and knotting techniques: comparative data. *Microsurgery* 2006; 26: 4-7.

2.   Miko I, Brath E, Furka I. Basic teaching in microsurgery. *Microsurgery* 2001; 21: 121-3.

58 D.

Myoglobinuria. Tissue/organ ischaemia causes complex patho-physiological processes depending on the duration and extent of the ischaemia. During reperfusion in the microcirculatory bed a 'no-reflow' phenomenon can be caused by microvascular spasm, swelling of endothelial cells, endothelial 'blebs', increased capillary permeability, interstitial oedema, microthrombi, plugged red blood cell aggregates, adhesion and plugging of neutrophil leukocytes, local acidosis and swollen myocytes around compressing vessels.

References

1.   Reffelmann T, Kloner RA. The 'no-reflow' phenomenon: basic science and clinical correlates. *Heart* 2002; 87: 162-8.

Section 2 questions

Hand surgery

1   The most frequent lesion found in obstetrical brachial plexus injuries involves:

A.   All cervical roots.
B.   Only C8 and T1.
C.   Only C6 and C7.
D.   Upper plexus C5, C6 and C7.
E.   Only C5.

2   The parents of a 2-week old boy bring the child to your clinic because he was born with a unilateral complete syndactyly of the thumb and the index finger. He has no other congenital abnormality. You examine the patient and order an X-ray that shows it to be a complex complete syndactyly of the first web space. You decide to:

A.   Wait until the child is 2 years of age or older to release the syndactyly without the need of a skin graft.
B.   Wait until the child is 4 years old and release the syndactyly using a split thickness skin graft.
C.   Wait for over 6 months and release the syndactyly under regional block to reduce the risk of anaesthesia and utilize a split thickness skin graft.
D.   Wait until the child is 3-6 months old and release the syndactyly using a full thickness skin graft from the groin.
E.   Wait until the child is 1-year-old and release the syndactyly with an open technique.

3 Correction of radial hand deformity is not indicated in patients that present:

A.   With thrombocytopenia with absent radius (TAR) syndrome.
B.   With Fanconi's anaemia.
C.   With Holt-Oram syndrome.
D.   As well-adapted adults.
E.   All of the above.

4 Which is not a test for thoracic outlet syndrome?

A.   Sunderland's.
B.   Roo's.
C.   Adson's.
D.   Morley's.
E.   Narakas.

5 Hypoplastic thumbs Type II of the Blauth classification can be treated successfully by:

A.   Releasing the contracted first web space, reconstruction of the ulnar collateral ligament, transposition flap to release the first web space, a full thickness skin graft and opponensplasty.
B.   Releasing the contracted first web space, reconstruction of the radial collateral ligament, transposition flap to release the first web space, a full thickness skin graft and opponensplasty.
C.   Amputation of the hypoplastic thumb and pollicisation of the index finger with use of a full thickness skin graft.
D.   Amputation of the hypoplastic thumb and pollicisation of the small finger with a split thickness skin graft.
E.   Amputation of the hypoplastic thumb and a toe-to-hand transfer.

6   In a fixed flexion contracture of the proximal interphalangeal (PIP) joint, the structure that is contributing most to the rigid flexion is:

A.   The collateral ligament.
B.   The contracted proximal part of the volar plate.
C.   The accessory collateral ligament.
D.   The rigid distal part of the volar plate.
E.   The flexor tendon.

7   Of the extensor tendon compartments on the dorsum of the wrist:

A.   The extensor pollicis longus (EPL) alters direction around the ulnar styloid.
B.   The extensor indicis proprius (EIP) shares a compartment with extensor digitorum communis (EDC).
C.   The first compartment contains the extensor carpi radialis longus (ECRL) and extensor carpi radialis brevis (ECRB).
D.   The posterior interosseous nerve runs in the third compartment.
E.   The extensor carpi ulnaris (ECU) and extensor digiti minimi (EDM) share the fifth compartment.

8   Of the bones in the carpus:

A.   The scaphoid is the largest bone.
B.   40% of the blood supply of the scaphoid enters via the waist of the bone.
C.   40% of the scaphoid surface is covered with articular cartilage.
D.   The kinetic forces of the carpus produce a tendency for the scaphoid to extend.
E.   Scapholunate dissociation is followed by flexion of the scaphoid.

9 The palmar aponeurosis:

A.   Covers the palm, including the central palm, thenar and hypothenar muscles.
B.   Is inserted into the flexor digitorum profundus tendons.
C.   Lies immediately deep to the neurovascular plane in the palm.
D.   Is inserted mainly into the bases of the proximal phalanges and the flexor sheaths.
E.   Consists of a direct extension of deep fascia of the forearm.

10 A contraindication to centralisation or radialisation of radial dysplasia is:

A.   Single extremity involvement.
B.   Stiff elbow.
C.   Stiff shoulder.
D.   Stiff fingers.
E.   Absent thumb.

11 Which nerve is not commonly used as a source of donor action in nerve transfer for treatment of brachial plexus injuries?

A.   Median nerve.
B.   Accessory nerve.
C.   Hypoglossal nerve.
D.   Ulnar nerve.
E.   Intercostal nerve

12 The 'safe' position of splintage of the hand includes:

A.   Metacarpophalangeal (MCP) joints straight.
B.   MCP joints flexed to approximately 60°.

C.   Proximal interphalangeal (PIP) joints flexed to approximately 90°.
D.   PIP joints flexed to approximately 60°.
E.   Distal interphalangeal (DIP) joints flexed to approximately 60°.

13 Of the vascular organisation in the hand:

A.   The collateral digital arteries in the finger arise from the superficial palmar arch.
B.   The collateral digital arteries arise from the deep palmar arch.
C.   The superficial palmar arch is usually complete, formed by contributions from the ulnar artery and radial arteries.
D.   The superficial palmar arch runs just superficial to the palmar aponeurosis.
E.   The deep palmar arch runs just deep to the palmar aponeurosis.

14 Of the major nerves in the forearm:

A.   The median nerve enters the forearm between the two heads of the supinator muscle.
B.   The posterior interosseous nerve enters the forearm between brachioradialis and extensor carpi radialis longus (ECRL).
C.   The anterior interosseous nerve runs on the interosseous membrane between flexor pollicis longus (FPL) and flexor digitorum profundus (FDP).
D.   The median nerve ends by supplying the wrist joint and no other more distal structure.
E.   The posterior interosseous nerve becomes purely cutaneous after supplying the forearm extensors.

15 The carpal tunnel:

A.   Contains the flexor carpi radialis (FCR).
B.   Contains the ulnar artery.
C.   Contains the flexor carpi ulnaris (FCU).
D.   Is formed by proximal and distal carpal rows and the flexor retinaculum.
E.   Shows no alteration in pressure on its contained structures in flexion or extension.

16 The initial event in the evolution of the development of a Boutonnière deformity is:

A. Lateral and palmar migration of extensor lateral bands.
B. Laxity or rupture of PIP joint volar plate.
C. Hyperextension of the DIP joint.
D. Loss of continuity of the central slip insertion into the back of the base of the middle phalanx.
E. Flexion contracture of the PIP joint.

17 In the correction of a swan neck deformity by operative procedure, it is essential to:

A. Repair the extensor mechanism on the dorsum of the PIP joint.
B. Achieve slight flexion or a neutral position of the PIP joint.
C. Divide the extensor mechanism distal to the PIP joint.
D. Release the volar plate.
E. Reef or tighten the central slip.

18 Of the lumbrical muscle, all statements are true except:

A. It has no attachment to bone.
B. It flexes the MCP joint.
C. It extends the PIP joint.
D. It is an abductor of the digit.
E. Paralysis leads to a claw hand.

19 Bilateral radial dysplasia with present thumbs of relative normal size is seen in association with:

A. Du Pan syndrome.
B. Holt-Oram syndrome.
C. Fanconi's anaemia.

D.   Clipperfield syndrome.
E.   TAR syndrome.

20 In the proximal row of the carpus, radiological signs of a ruptured scapholunate ligament include all but:

A.   A wide gap between the scaphoid and lunate.
B.   A flexed scaphoid.
C.   An extended scaphoid.
D.   An extended lunate.
E.   A flexed triquetral.

21 In thumb hypoplasia, classified by Blauth, all these statements are true except:

A.   Blauth 1 generally requires no active treatment other than consideration of an opponensplasty.
B.   Surgery for Blauth 2 may require stabilisation of a lax MCP joint.
C.   The crucial element determining management of Blauth 3 is the state of development of the basal carpometacarpal (CMC) joint.
D.   The standard management of Blauth 4 is reinforcement of the hypoplastic thumb by bone stabilisation and tendon transfer.
E.   Blauth 5 may be associated with radial ray anomalies.

22 In the finger, what is the usual relationship of the digital nerve to the digital artery?

A.   Dorsal.
B.   Volar.
C.   Proximal.
D.   Distal.
E.   Lateral.

23 Contraindications to early exploration in brachial plexus injury include:

A. Presence of Horner's syndrome.
B. Absence of a Tinel's sign in the supraclavicular fossa.
C. Presence of a separate skeletal injury.
D. Presence of root avulsion on MRI.
E. Injury caused by a gunshot.

24 In older patients with traumatic amputation of the thumb, when you perform a pollicisation, surgical intervention differs from young children with congenital absent thumbs in that:

A. In traumatic cases of older patients it is necessary to shorten the flexor tendons.
B. In traumatic cases of older patients it is necessary to use a bone graft to replace the missing metacarpal.
C. In younger patients the extensor tendons do not need shortening.
D. In older patients the extensor tendons do not need shortening.
E. In congenital cases it is always necessary to utilize a full thickness skin graft.

25 Toe-to-hand transfer in patients with bilateral hands affected with constriction ring syndrome:

A. Should not be performed as there is no cortical representation for the missing part of the hand.
B. Should be performed in cases of painful tip of the digits to provide padding to the end of the digits and required length.
C. Do not have any function because of lack of motion.
D. Always require a tendon and nerve graft.
E. Have a high probability of failure because the arteries are not well developed.

26 In radial dysplasia:

A. The ulna physis can tolerate degloving and devascularisation.
B. The ulna is usually affected.
C. The ulna is fused to the carpus in centralisation.
D. Recurrence of the deformity is unusual if radialisation is properly performed.
E. Distraction lengthening of the ulna should be performed pre-operatively.

27 Poor results in the treatment of radial club hand are due to:

A. Inadequate pre-operative stretching.
B. Improper surgical technique.
C. No compliance with postoperative bracing.
D. Centralisation in patients with a stiff elbow.
E. All of the above.

28 Fanconi pancytopenia includes:

A. Mental retardation.
B. Short stature.
C. Brown pigment of the skin.
D. Kidney malformation.
E. All of the above.

29 In radial dysplasia - utilizing the Ilizarov system, limb lengthening is associated with:

A. Elbow pain and stiffness of all digits.
B. Night pain and delayed union of the callus.
C. Pin tract infection.
D. A and C.
E. All of the above.

30 Rupture of the C5 and C6 roots will paralyze which group of muscles?

A. Subclavius and infraspinatus.
B. Deltoid and teres minor.
C. Supraspinatus and brachioradialis.
D. Biceps brachii and brachialis.
E. All of the above.

31 In obstetrical brachial plexus paralysis, root avulsion of C5 and C6 with an inability to flex the elbow can be treated with success and no obvious morbidity by which nerve transfer?

A. 10% axillary nerve to musculocutaneous.
B. 10% lateral cord to musculocutaneous.
C. 10% of ulnar nerve to musculocutaneous.
D. 10% of radial nerve to musculocutaneous.
E. All of the above.

32 In radial dysplasia:

A. Radialisation involves resection of a portion of the carpus.
B. Radialisation involves tendon transfers of radial tendons to create an ulnar balancing force.
C. Release of the ulnar anlage may prevent deterioration.
D. Re-distribution of the skin can be done by Z-plasties.
E. Pollicisation should be done before the radialisation.

33 Which is correct in relation to replantation of a digit?

A. Is not advisable at the DIP joint level.
B. Should only be considered with guillotine injuries.
C. Is generally not recommended for proximal Urbaniak Class III ring avulsion/amputation injuries.

D.   Is not successful when cold ischaemia exceeds 24 hours.
E.   Is more successful with postoperative IV heparin.

34 In nerve transfer for brachial plexus injury:

A.   The intercostal nerves are often transferred to the median nerve.
B.   The phrenic nerve cannot be used because of the risk of respiratory compromise.
C.   The spinal accessory nerve causes complete paralysis of trapezius.
D.   The axillary nerve can be innervated by the nerves to triceps.
E.   The contralateral plexus is never used.

35 A 43-year-old woman has a pinpoint area of tenderness at the base of the nail of the left ring finger. The area is painful to touch and sensitive to cold. Physical examination of the finger shows a deformity of the nail plate. Which of the following is the most likely diagnosis?

A.   Epidermal inclusion cyst.
B.   Ganglion cyst.
C.   Giant cell tumour.
D.   Glomus tumour.
E.   Neurilemmoma.

36 In obstetrical brachial plexus palsy:

A.   The incidence has declined over the last 50 years due to more intensive obstetric intervention.
B.   Shoulder dystocia is associated with over 90% of cases.
C.   Other important associated factors are assisted delivery and low birth weight.
D.   The incidence is higher in breech delivery.
E.   A differential diagnosis includes shoulder injury, cervical cord lesions and arthrogryphosis.

37 Arthritis can be treated by all except:

A.   Joint excision.
B.   Joint mobilisation under anaesthesia.
C.   Joint osteotomy.
D.   Joint fusion.
E.   Denervation.

38 In De Quervain's tenosynovitis (tenovaginitis) all are true except:

A.   Can be assessed by Finkelstein's test.
B.   Can be assessed by Eichoff's test.
C.   False positive tests can occur in radial neuritis.
D.   Steroid injection and splintage are better than either alone.
E.   Multiple slips of both abductor pollicis longus (APL) and extensor pollicis brevis (EPB) can be present.

39 In Dupuytren's disease:

A.   Splinting may prevent progression of the contracture.
B.   Is more strongly associated with alcohol than smoking.
C.   Has a genetic basis linked to chromosome 17.
D.   Fasciotomy has equal recurrence rates as fasciectomy.
E.   Needle fasciotomy is as successful in correcting MCP joint contracture as fasciectomy.

40 Regarding tumours in the hand:

A.   Hildreth's test differentiates glomus tumours from other vascular tumours.
B.   Giant cell tumours of tendon sheath recur commonly and are usually benign.
C.   Giant cell tumours of tendon sheath are always related to synovium.
D.   Melorheostosis is a lymphoma.
E.   Melanoma does not occur on the hand.

41 Infection can be mimicked by all except:

A.   Pigmented villonodular synovioma.
B.   Calcific tendonitis.
C.   Epithelioid sarcoma.
D.   Osteoid osteoma.
E.   Reflex sympathetic dystrophy (RSD)/chronic regional pain syndrome (CRPS).

42 Signs or tests associated with glomus tumours include the following except:

A.   Love.
B.   Hildreth.
C.   Soucquet-Hoyer.
D.   Ethyl alcohol.
E.   Cherry red mass.

43 The least common sarcoma in the hand:

A.   Chondrosarcoma.
B.   Epithelioid.
C.   Liposarcoma.
D.   Fibrosarcoma.
E.   Synovial sarcoma.

44 One of the following is not an accepted theory of the aetiology of ganglia:

A.   Ball valve.
B.   Embryonic rest.
C.   Myxoid degeneration.
D.   Traumatic perforation.
E.   Neurovascular channels.

45 The following is true of epithelioid sarcoma except:

A.   May present as Dupuytren's disease.
B.   May mimic infection.
C.   May mimic melanoma.
D.   Spreads to lymph nodes.
E.   Sentinel lymph node biopsy confers staging benefit.

46 In carpal tunnel syndrome which is false?

A.   There is a 25% incidence in males.
B.   Carpal tunnel decompression was first performed in 1896.
C.   It is commonly bilateral.
D.   The motor branch is vulnerable as it passes through the transverse carpal ligament in up to 25% of cases.
E.   The age of presentation rises towards a peak in the late fifties.

47 Common locations for compression of the ulnar nerve include all except:

A.   Ligament of Struthers.
B.   Medial intermuscular septum.
C.   Osbourne's canal.
D.   Between the two heads of flexor carpi ulnaris (FCU).
E.   The deep FCU aponeurosis.

48 The following is true of the ulnar nerve in Guyon's canal except:

A.   Compression in the first part results in sensory and motor palsy.
B.   Compression in the third part results in sensory symptoms only.
C.   Compression in the first portion of the second part results in motor symptoms only.
D.   Can cause Ramsay Hunt syndrome.
E.   The second part of Guyon's canal starts at the hamate.

49 Which of the following are not differentials for nerve compression neuropathies?

A. Hereditary neuropathy with liability to pressure palsies.
B. Tomaculous neuropathy.
C. Neuralgic amyotrophy.
D. Multifocal motor neuropathy.
E. Charcot Marie Tooth.

50 Symbrachydactyly:

A. On the right is associated with Poland's syndrome.
B. Is rarely confused with constriction ring syndrome.
C. Falls under failure of formation in the International Federation of Societies for Surgery of the Hand (IFSSH) classification.
D. Can be treated by pollicisation.
E. Often has transverse lying bones.

51 The following are primary causes of mono-neuropathy except:

A. Entrapment.
B. Osteoarthritis.
C. Ischaemia.
D. Tumours.
E. Hypothyroidism.

52 The following are infectious causes of mono-neuropathies except:

A. Lyme disease.
B. Leprosy.
C. Herpes zoster.
D. Bilharzia (schistosomiasis).
E. Diphtheria.

53 Hereditary neuropathy with liability to pressure palsies is associated with all, except:

A.   Familial predisposition.
B.   Interstitial deletion in chromosome 17p11.2-12.
C.   Defect in gene for central nerve axonal transport.
D.   Spontaneous recovery.
E.   Hereditary motor and sensory neuropathy.

54 The presence of eyelid ptosis and pupillary miosis known as Horner syndrome may be noted in obstetric brachial plexus paralysis, suggesting:

A.   Upper trunk rupture.
B.   Phrenic nerve palsy.
C.   Avulsion of the lower brachial plexus.
D.   C5, C6 and C7 avulsion.
E.   All of the above.

55 Amniotic Band syndrome is associated with all except:

A.   Patterson's classification.
B.   Peripheral neuropathy.
C.   Constriction rings.
D.   Ectodermal necrosis aetiological theory.
E.   Lymphoedema.

56 Thumb hypoplasias are frequently associated with:

A.   Scaphoid anomalies.
B.   Weckesser's classification.
C.   Toe transfers.

D.   Mandatory surgical reconstruction.
E.   First web space tightness.

57 In pollicisation:

A.   The metacarpal head becomes the new trapezium.
B.   The distal phalanx becomes the new proximal phalanx.
C.   The optimal position is for the new trapezium to lie lateral to the trapezoid.
D.   The first dorsal interosseous becomes a thumb adductor.
E.   The extensor tendon should not be split beyond the level of the MCP joint.

58 In thumb duplication:

A.   Always reconstruct the ulnar collateral ligament of the MCP joint.
B.   Always excise the triphalangeal thumb.
C.   Always look for pollex abductus.
D.   Cloquet described the excision and combination of two halves of the thumbs to make one thumb before Bilhaut.
E.   Always needs treatment.

59 The treatment of choice for a Blauth grade 3b hypoplastic thumb would be:

A.   Toe transfer.
B.   Pollicisation.
C.   Reconstruction of CMC and tendon transfers.
D.   Huber-Nicolayasen transfer.
E.   Distraction lengthening.

60 In a typical cleft hand:

A.   There are finger nubbins.
B.   Usually involves the left hand.
C.   Is associated with autosomal dominant inheritance.
D.   Usually has a good thumb.
E.   Function is poor.

61 In radial dysplasia:

A.   The radial nerve can be large.
B.   The ECRB/L are available for transfer.
C.   The median artery can be persistent.
D.   The extensor carpi ulnaris (ECU) is shortened.
E.   The carpus is subluxed volarly.

62 In polydactyly, the following is true except:

A.   Stelling Type A can be treated by ligation.
B.   Ligation leaves a nubbin.
C.   Reconstruction of the ulnar collateral ligament is necessary.
D.   Is associated with Ellis van Creveld and Lawrence Moon Bardet Biedl syndromes.
E.   Can be hereditary.

63 Which one of the following components of a limb allograft will elicit the most and the least cellular immune response following transplantation?

A.   Skin and muscle.
B.   Skin and subcutaneous tissue.
C.   Muscle and bone.
D.   Muscle and vessel.
E.   Skin and vessel.

64 Giant cell tumours are associated with all except:

A. Pigmented villonodular synovioma.
B. Localised or diffuse presentations.
C. Pigmentation.
D. Haemosiderin.
E. Exclusively synovial origins.

65 In replantation of an avulsed thumb:

A. Avoid shortening the bone.
B. Flexor pollicis longus (FPL) function should be restored.
C. The thumb should be supinated rather than pronated.
D. A vein graft from the radial artery in the anatomical snuffbox is often necessary.
E. Arteries are more resistant to intimal damage than veins.

66 In hand embryology:

A. The apical ectodermal ridge governs thumb development.
B. The apical ectodermal ridge secretes fibroblast derived growth factor 4.
C. The apical ectodermal ridge influences the *sonic hedgehog* gene.
D. Wnt-7a is expressed by the apical ectodermal ridge.
E. The apical ectodermal ridge controls the dorsal-ventral axis.

67 The most common form of carpal instability is:

A. Midcarpal instability.
B. Scapholunate instability.
C. Lunotriquetral instability.
D. Peritrapezoid instability.
E. Transtrapezial instability.

68 In arthrogryphosis:

A.   The arms should be positioned one up and one down.
B.   Wedge osteotomy of the carpus can improve the hand position.
C.   The arms may benefit from internal rotation osteotomies.
D.   The aetiology is related to muscular dystrophy.
E.   Intelligence is often sub-normal.

69 DeQuervain's stenosing tenosynovitis is most often clinically confused with:

A.   Carpal tunnel syndrome.
B.   Lunatomalacia.
C.   Dupuytren's contracture.
D.   Osteoarthritis of the CMC joint of the thumb.
E.   An interosseous ganglion of the scaphoid.

70 Regarding syndactyly:

A.   Web creep is less likely to occur if the separation is performed after age two.
B.   Is associated with maternal diabetes.
C.   Classification includes shovel hand.
D.   Causes no functional problems.
E.   Is the commonest congenital hand condition.

71 In the surgical treatment of trigger finger, what structure is incised?

A.   The A1 pulley alone.
B.   The A2 pulley.
C.   Both the A1 pulley and usually (not necessarily intentionally) the C2 pulley.
D.   The A4 pulley.
E.   Both Grayson's ligament and the A1 pulley.

72 The following is true of congenital upper limb anomalies except:

A. They are commonly sub-classified according to thumb status.
B. The teratologic sequence of Ogino includes clefting, symbrachydactyly and polydactyly.
C. They occur in 1:150 births.
D. Swanson's IFSSH classification attempts to relate the embryological origin of the anomalies.
E. They are likely to be bilateral in 50%.

73 The middle finger extension test (active extension against resistance) is useful for all except:

A. Intrinsic tightness.
B. Radial tunnel syndrome.
C. Carpal pathology.
D. Multifocal motor neuropathy.
E. Posterior interosseous nerve palsy.

74 In rheumatoid arthritis:

A. Anti-TNF alpha prevents articular destruction and tendon rupture.
B. Rheumatoid nodules can be treated successfully by intra-lesional steroids.
C. A positive response to rheumatoid disease modifying agents is one of the diagnostic features.
D. Thumb surgery is considered a low-risk, high-benefit procedure.
E. Correction of ulnar drift should precede correction of wrist pathology.

75 Which one of the following is a diagnostic criterion for rheumatoid arthritis according to the American Academy of Rheumatology?

A. Arthritis of the hand for >6 weeks.
B. Morning stiffness for 2 weeks.
C Positive pANCA or cANCA antibodies.
D. Normocytic anaemia.
E. Typical ocular changes (scleritis, episcleritis).

76 In Dupuytren's disease:

A. There is an increased ratio of Type I to Type III collagen.
B. There is an increased ratio of Type II to Type III collagen.
C. There is an increased ratio of Type III to Type I collagen.
D. There is an increased ratio of Type III to Type IV collagen.
E. There is an increased ratio of Type II to Type I collagen.

77 The commonest inheritance pattern for Dupuytren's disease is:

A. Autosomal recessive.
B. Autosomal dominant.
C. Sporadic.
D. Sex-linked dominant.
E. Sex-linked recessive.

78 The following is the commonest cause of distal interphalangeal joint contracture in Dupuytren's disease:

A. Spiral band.
B. Lateral digital sheet.
C. Pre-tendinous cord.
D. Retrovascular cord of Thomine.
E. Spiral cord.

79 Absolute indications for surgery in Dupuytren's disease include:

A. Painless Garrod's pads.
B. Plantar nodules.
C. Any contracture of the MCP joint.
D. Any contracture of the PIP joint.
E. None of the above.

80 Concerning carpal tunnel syndrome - all are true except:

A. The radial border of the carpal tunnel is the scaphoid and ridge of trapezium.
B. The ulnar border is the hook of the hamate and the pisiform bone.
C. Conduction velocity can improve within 2 weeks of decompression.
D. The sensitivity of nerve conduction studies is over 80%.
E. The specificity of nerve conduction studies is less than 70%.

81 Regarding rehabilitation of tendon injuries:

A. A volar slab is best for flexor tendon injuries.
B. A dorsal slab in extension is best for flexor tendon injuries.
C. Klienert traction is reserved for thumb injuries.
D. The Belfast regime is a 'CAM' regime, i.e. controlled active motion.
E. Immobilisation for 4 weeks is proven to increase the success of tenolysis.

82 A Stener lesion occurs when:

A. The ulnar collateral ligament is obstructed by the abductor pollicis brevis (APB).
B. The ulnar collateral ligament is obstructed by extensor pollicis longus (EPL).

C. The ulnar collateral ligament is obstructed by extensor pollicis brevis (EPB).
D. The ulnar collateral ligament is obstructed by the adductor pollicis aponeurosis.
E. The ulnar collateral ligament is obstructed by abductor pollicis longus (APL).

83 The most appropriate angles for fusion of the digits are:

A. Index - 5° DIP joint, 40° PIP joint, 25° MCP joint.
B. Index - 10° DIP joint, 10° PIP joint, neutral MCP joint.
C. Thumb - neutral IP joint, neutral MCP joint.
D. Thumb - neutral IP joint, 45° MCP joint.
E. Little finger - neutral DIP joint, neutral PIP joint, neutral MCP joint.

Section 2 answers

Hand surgery

1 D.

Upper plexus C5, C6 and C7.

References

1. Hentz VR. Obstetric brachial plexus palsy. In: *Plastic Surgery*. Mathes D, Ed; Hentz VR, Volume Editor. Saunders Elsevier, 2006.

2. Smith NC, Rowan P, Benson LJ, Ezaki M, Carter PR. Neonatal brachial plexus palsy outcome of absent biceps function at three months of age. *J Bone Joint Surg [Am]* 2004; 86(10): 2163-70.

2 D.

Wait until the child is 3-6 months old and release the syndactyly using a full thickness skin graft from the groin. Release of syndactyly of unequal length digits should be performed as early as possible; between 3 and 6 months is a good time as the child is old enough to withstand the procedure without undue anaesthetic risk, whilst the chances of damage to the joints are reduced, especially the PIP joint of the longer digit. If the procedure is delayed the child will develop permanent changes to the PIP joint. Syndactyly is more common in males, is present bilaterally in 50% of affected patients, and often is associated with other musculoskeletal malformations or systemic syndromes. The goal of syndactyly release is to create a functional hand with the fewest surgical procedures while minimising complications. For simple syndactyly, surgical reconstruction can begin at approximately 6 months, although many surgeons prefer to wait until the infant is 18 months old. Special situations, such as complex syndactyly and involvement of border digits, may warrant surgical intervention earlier than 6 months. Reconstruction of the web commissure is the most technically challenging part of the operation, followed by separation of the remaining digits. Full thickness skin grafting is almost always required for soft-tissue coverage. Complex syndactyly and syndactyly associated with other hand anomalies warrant special consideration. After reconstruction, patients should be examined periodically until they have achieved skeletal maturity because late complications such as web creep can occur.

References

1.   Dao KD, Shin AY, Billings A, Oberg KC, Wood VE. Surgical treatment of congenital syndactyly of the hand. *J Am Acad Orthop Surg* 2004; 12(1): 39-48.

3   D.

As well-adapted adults. Adults well adjusted to the use of their radial dysplastic hand are not candidates for surgical reconstruction as they are able to perform all the activities of daily living with the hand as it is. Bayne outlined five categories of patients in which treatment is contraindicated: 1) patients with minimal anomalies; 2) patients with severe associated anomalies, who have severe retardation, poor prognosis and short predicted lifespan; 3) adult or older patients, who have adjusted to the disability and have acquired dexterity in performing activities of daily living; 4) patients with stiff elbows in which the straightened hand will not be able to reach the mouth or the perineum; and, 5) patients with severe soft tissue contractures that also involve the neurovascular structures.

References

1.   Dobyns JH, Wood VE, Bayne LG. Congenital hand deformities. In: *Operative hand surgery*, Vol 1, 3rd ed. Green DP, Ed. New York, USA: Churchill Livingstone; 1993: 288-303.

2.   Bayne LG. Radial deficiencies. In: *Reconstruction of the child's hand*. Carter PR, Ed. New York, USA: Lea and Febiger; 1991: 187-97.

4 A.

Sunderland's. Sunderland's test is not a described test.

5 A.

Releasing the contracted first web space, reconstruction of the ulnar collateral ligament, transposition flap to release the first web space, a full thickness skin graft and opponensplasty. In hypoplasia of the thumb, Blauth Type 2, the thumb is smaller and less stable than normal. The hypoplasia has three elements: 1) adduction contracture of the first web space is apparent because of 2) the lack of thenar muscles, and the hand compensates by exhibiting 3) laxity of the ulnar collateral ligament that allows abduction of the MCP joint. The skeleton, although small, has normal articulations. Treatment of this condition requires: a) release of the first web space using a dorsal flap from the thumb - preferably, as described by Strauch, and closing the thumb defect with a full thickness skin graft; b) reconstruction of the ulnar collateral ligament, as described by Lister using the division of the flexor digitorum superficialis (FDS) that is utilized for c) an opponensplasty, as described by Royle. There are other methods for soft tissue release, ligament reconstruction and opponensplasty, but this is the simplest and probably the least invasive while reducing morbidity of donor sites.

References

1. Strauch B. Dorsal thumb flap for release of adduction contracture of the first web space. *Bull Hosp Joint Dis* 1975; 36(1): 34-9.

2. Lister G. *The hand: diagnosis and indications*, 2nd ed. London, UK: Churchill Livingstone; 1984: 312-51.

3. Royle ND. An operation for paralysis of the intrinsic muscles of the thumb. *JAMA* 1938; 111: 612.

6 B.

The contracted proximal part of the volar plate. When the PIP joint flexes, the flexible proximal part of the volar plate (the check reins) folds back on itself to permit flexion. Left in this position, the folded portions adhere to each other and contract. This is the articular element that contracts and rigidly prevents extension.

7 B.

The extensor indicis proprius (EIP) shares a compartment with extensor digitorum communis (EDC). The first compartment contains APL and EPB. The second compartment contains ECRL and ECRB. The third compartment contains EPL altering direction around the tubercle of Lister. The fourth compartment contains EDC, EIP and the posterior interosseous nerve. The fifth compartment contains EDM. The sixth compartment contains ECU.

8 E.

Scapholunate dissociation is followed by flexion of the scaphoid. The capitate is the largest of the carpal bones. 80% of the scaphoid blood supply enters at the waist (hence the predilection to non-union of a proximal pole fracture) and 80% of the scaphoid surface is covered in articular cartilage. The kinetic forces of the carpus produce a tendency for the scaphoid to flex. The scaphoid moves into flexion if it is released from the lunate by laxity or rupture of the scapholunate ligament.

9 D.

Is inserted mainly into the bases of the proximal phalanges and the flexor sheaths. The palmar aponeurosis is phylogenetically the degenerated, flattened, distal part of the tendon of palmaris longus, a weak flexor of the long digits, by virtue of its insertion into the bases of the proximal phalanges and the fibrous flexor sheaths. (It also inserts into the deep transverse metacarpal ligament and some fibres extend distally along the digit). The aponeurosis is immediately superficial to the neurovascular structures in the central palm, anchoring the skin, and does not extend over the thenar or hypothenar muscles, which are freer to alter shape.

10 B.

Stiff elbow. A stiff elbow is a contraindication for centralisation or radialisation of the radial club hand as the centralised hand will not be able to reach the mouth or the perineum when the elbow does not have flexion passing 90°.

References

1.   Dobyns JH, Wood VE, Bayne LG. Congenital hand deformities. In: *Operative hand surgery*, Vol 1, 3rd ed. Green DP, Ed. New York, USA: Churchill Livingstone; 1993: 288-303.

2.   Bayne LG. Radial deficiencies. In: *Reconstruction of the child's hand.* Carter PR, Ed. New York, USA: Lea and Febiger; 1991: 187-97.

11 C.

Hypoglossal nerve. Historically the hypoglossal nerve was used as a nerve transfer in brachial plexus palsy but it is not used in modern surgery. Fascicles from the median nerve and also the ulnar nerve are often used to innervate the motor branches to brachialis and biceps in the arm. Usually the fascicles of the ulnar nerve identified as innervating FCU are used to neurotise the motor branches to biceps (Oberlin's transfer). Similarly, the flexor carpi radialis (FCR) fascicles from the median nerve can be used to neurotise the motor nerve to brachialis. Intercostal nerves are also a useful source of motor axons. The intercostal nerves can be transferred, if possible without nerve grafts, to the musculocutaneous nerve, the nerves to triceps, the thoracodorsal nerve or the long thoracic nerve. They can also be used to neurotise the motor nerves of muscles used in free muscle transfer.

12 B.

MCP joints flexed to approximately 60°. The safe position of splintage of any joint is that in which the maximum number of ligaments are at maximum tension (the 'close packed' position). The CAM shape of the metacarpal head produces maximum tension in the collateral ligaments in flexion.

Flexion of the PIP joint produces folding of the proximal (flexible) part of the volar ligament, which rapidly contracts and a flexion contracture results. The DIP joint ligaments are maximally tense in extension. The safe position for splintage of the hand includes MCP joint flexion, with PIP and DIP joints in full extension.

13 A.

The collateral digital arteries in the finger arise from the superficial palmar arch. The superficial palmar arch, usually incomplete, is the direct continuation of the ulnar artery. In a minority of hands, this arch is completed by a contribution from a branch of the radial artery. It runs just deep to the palmar aponeurosis and gives off the collateral 'true' digital arteries. The deep palmar arch is more usually complete and is formed by the terminal branch of the radial artery and a contribution from the ulnar artery. It lies deep in the palm, immediately superficial to the metacarpals.

14 C.

The anterior interosseous nerve runs on the interosseous membrane between flexor pollicis longus (FPL) and flexor digitorum profundus (FDP). The median nerve enters the forearm between the two heads of pronator teres. It ends by supplying the thenar muscles and the skin of the radial digits, including the pulps. The posterior interosseous nerve enters the extensor compartment between the two heads of supinator and ends by supplying the wrist joint, without cutaneous distribution. The anterior interosseous nerve leaves the median nerve in the proximal forearm and runs in the interosseous membrane between FPL and FDP, supplying both.

15 D.

Is formed by proximal and distal carpal rows and the flexor retinaculum. It transmits the median nerve, and nine flexor tendons: the FPL and two to each long digit. The ulnar artery overlies the ulnar border of the flexor retinaculum, outside the carpal tunnel. The FCU travels outside the tunnel, inserting, via the pisiform bone, piso-hamate and piso-metacarpal ligaments into the ulnar carpus. The FCR lies in its own tunnel, in the groove beneath the ridge of trapezium, distinct from the main carpal tunnel cavity. Pressure in the carpal tunnel rises with each degree movement away from neutral (0°).

16 D.

Loss of continuity of the central slip insertion into the back of the base of the middle phalanx. The initial event in the development of a Boutonnière deformity is loss of continuity of the central slip insertion into the back of the middle phalanx base. This is followed by dissociation of the central slip from the lateral bands and palmar migration of the lateral slips until they go past the axis of the joint and become flexors. The back of the joint 'buttonholes' through the extensor mechanism. This position rapidly becomes fixed. The lateral slips now act entirely on the DIP joint producing hyperextension. Rigid flexion contracture of the PIP joint is a secondary, non-specific outcome of prolonged flexion of this joint.

17 B.

Achieve slight flexion or a neutral position of the PIP joint. The determining event in development of a swan neck deformity is hyperextension at the level of the PIP joint. This can be secondary to an uncorrected mallet deformity (when the long extensors, unable to extend the DIP joint, over-extend the PIP joint), malunion in extension of a fracture around the PIP joint, or loss of flexing forces at the PIP joint, the volar plate and the FDS being the main factors. All conservative or operative methods of swan neck correction include, as an essential feature, correction of the PIP joint to neutral or slight flexion.

18 D.

It is an abductor of the digit. This statement is incorrect; the lumbrical has no attachment to bone. It arises from the tendon of FDP and inserts into the long extensor complex. The lumbrical flexes the MCP joint and extends the PIP joint. Paralysis results in the opposite of such actions, the claw posture (or 'intrinsic minus position'), which consists of a hyperextended MCP joint and a flexed PIP joint. The lumbrical has no radial deviation vector on the digit.

19 E.

TAR syndrome. Thrombocytopenia-absent radius (TAR) syndrome is an autosomal recessive disorder characterised by congenital thrombocytopenia, leukocytosis and bilateral total aplasia of the radius with present thumbs. Although the thumb in TAR syndrome patients is of relatively normal size and shape, it is held in a position of MCP flexion in most patients and function is impaired.

References

1.   Goldfarb CA, Wustrack R, Pratt JA, Mender A, Manske PR. Thumb function and appearance in thrombocytopenia-absent radius syndrome. *J Hand Surg [Am]* 2007; 32(2): 157-61.

20 C.

An extended scaphoid. A wide gap between scaphoid and lunate is otherwise known as the Terry Thomas sign in reference to a British actor with a gap in his teeth. A flexed scaphoid leads to the signet ring sign on plain radiography. The radiological gap between scaphoid and lunate should be equal to that of other intercarpal joint spaces. The kinetics of the carpus produces a strong tendency for the scaphoid to flex and the triquetral to extend, with the lunate linking these two conflicting forces. Dissociaton between the scaphoid and lunate permits the scaphoid to flex, while the lunate, under the pull of the triquetrum, via the luno-triquetral ligament, extends (dorsal intercalated segment instability [DISI]).

21 D.

The standard management of Blauth 4 is reinforcement of the hypoplastic thumb by bone stabilisation and tendon transfer. This statement is incorrect; the standard management of Blauth 4 is NOT reinforcement of the hypoplastic thumb by bone stabilisation and tendon transfer. Blauth 1 describes a mildly hypoplastic thumb with hypoplastic or absent short thenar muscles. Opposition is weak or absent. Blauth 2 often includes laxity of the MCP joint and the ulnar collateral ligament requires reinforcement. Blauth 3 contains a variable development of the CMC joint. In essence, a good CMC joint leaves a potentially useful thumb, capable of reinforcement by tendon transfers; a poor CMC joint is likely to dictate a pollicisation. Blauth 4 describes the 'pouce flottant' or floating thumb. This is generally of no functional use and standard management includes its removal and a pollicisation. Blauth 5 describes total absence of the thumb with variable associated anomalies of the entire radial ray.

22 B.

Volar. In the digit the digital nerves usually lie medial and slightly volar to the digital arteries.

23 B.

Absence of a Tinel's sign in the supraclavicular fossa. The following is a contraindication to early exploration in brachial plexus injury. There are advocates for immediate exploration of brachial plexus injuries and also advocates for delayed exploration. When there is a strong suspicion of root avulsion and nerve rupture, surgical exploration is without doubt warranted at an early stage. Horner's syndrome is strongly correlated with avulsion of C8/T1 roots. It is a poor prognostic sign for spontaneous recovery. Presence of a Tinel's sign in the supraclavicular region indicates a post-ganglionic injury, and thus a possibility of recovery. Absence of a Tinel's sign may indicate a preganglionic injury and thus is a bad prognostic sign indicating early exploration. The presence of a pseudomeningocele on MRI indicates root avulsion and again is a factor indicating early exploration. Fracture of the first rib and injury caused by gunshot are both high-energy injuries that would indicate significant trauma to the plexus and again warrant early exploration.

24 A.

In traumatic cases of older patients it is necessary to shorten the flexor tendons. When pollicisation is performed in children at the age of 6 months, only the extensor mechanism needs to be tightened. As the child grows, doubling in size over the next 6 months, the flexor tendons become active without the need for surgery. This avoids surgery to the flexors and resultant scarring. In older children, the growth is not so remarkably fast and it is necessary to shorten the flexor mechanism during the surgery for pollicisation since the child is also more dependent on the use of both hands than the infant.

References

1.   Scheker LR, Cendales LC. Correcting congenital thumb anomalies in children: opponensplasty and pollicization. In: *The growing hand: diagnosis and management of the upper extremity in children.* Gupta A, Kay SPJ, Scheker LR. St. Louis, USA: Mosby, 2000: 171-82.

25 B.

Should be performed in cases of painful tip of the digits to provide padding to the end of the digits and required length. Children with constriction ring syndrome often have multiple digits involved and therefore a cross finger flap is not an option. Toe-to-hand transfer brings not only length but sensation and a stable tip and is especially important in cases in which the tip of a particular finger is painful with an ischaemic tip because of skin shortage.

Toe-to-hand transfer is a well-established reconstructive option for certain congenital hand anomalies [1]. It is the only technique which can add growth potential to the immature skeleton. Toe transfer is best suited for constriction ring amputations, which have relatively normal proximal anatomy. Transfers should be performed early in life to avoid lack of cortical integration of the new part. Anatomic variations of both hand and foot are often encountered, which influence both operative approach and functional prognosis. Constriction ring syndrome is classified by Patterson into: I - a simple band; II - a construction band with distal lymphoedema; III - with acrosyndactyly; and IV - congenital amputation.

References

1.   Eaton CJ, Lister, GD. Toe transfer for congenital hand defects. *Microsurgery* 1991; 12(3): 186-95.

26 B.

The ulna is usually affected. It is frequently short and radially bowed.

27 E.

All of the above. The treatment of radial dysplasia (previously called club hand) includes a team effort in which the parents or guardian play an important role in the success of the treatment, by stretching the soft tissue with passive exercises and postoperatively making sure the patient wears an adequate brace to maintain the correction until the skeleton is fully mature. Selecting patients for surgical intervention is the first step in achieving good and excellent results.

References

1.   Bayne LG, Klug MS. Long-term review of the surgical treatment of radial deficiencies. *J Hand Surg [Am]* 1987; 12(2): 169-79.

28 E.

All of the above. Fanconi anaemia was described for the first time in 1927. It is an autosomal recessive disease that presents as a progressive pancytopenia, usually late in the first decade of life, in association with multiple anomalies (Table 1).

Table 1. Fanconi anaemia and associated multiple anomalies.	
Anomaly	**Occurrence %**
Abnormal pigmentation	75
Skeletal deformities	59
Growth retardation	56
Microcephaly	43
Renal anomalies	28
Strabismus	26
Hypogonadism	22
Mental retardation	21

References

1.   Tarantino MD, Kline RM. Hematologic disorders and the hand. In: *The growing hand: diagnosis and management of the upper extremity in children*. Gupta A, Kay SPJ, Scheker LR. St. Louis, USA: Mosby, 2000: 401-14.

29 E.

All of the above. Children affected with radial dysplasia have a tendency to have stiff fingers with marked hypoplasia from radial to ulnar, the index finger is less developed than the small finger and on occasion the small finger is bigger than the index and middle fingers. The muscles are short and the median nerve runs on the radial aspect of the forearm under considerable tension. Lengthening of the forearm makes the median nerve even tighter and the fingers stiffer.

In a study on radial dysplasia and limb lengthening, six children with radial dysplasia had distraction lengthening of the ulna. The mean lengthening achieved was 4.7cm (46% of original ulna length). Complications included nocturnal pain, pin tract infection and callus fracture or delayed union. Distraction lengthening of the ulna facilitated activities of daily living, such as reaching the perineum or driving, but at the cost of an increased complication rate. The high rate of callus fractures highlighted the need for regular radiographic review during distraction and suggests that after distraction it may take more than 4 weeks for satisfactory callus consolidation before removal of the fixator.

References

1.   Pickford MA, Scheker LR. Distraction lengthening of the ulna in radial club hand using the Ilizarov technique. *J Hand Surg [Br]* 1998; 23(2): 186-91.

30   E.

All of the above.

References

1.   Durrant DH, True JM, Blum JW. *Myelopathy, radiculopathy, and peripheral entrapment syndromes.* Florida, USA: CRC Press, 2002: 347 appendix.

2.   http://anatomy.uams.edu/anatomyhtml/nerves_upperlimb.html.

31   C.

10% of ulnar nerve to musculocutaneous. Upper brachial plexus avulsion injuries cause impairment of shoulder and elbow function which is very disabling for patients. Restoration of elbow flexion is the first goal to be achieved in order to restore arm function. In cases of nerve root rupture, the majority show successful results after repair, but in nerve root avulsions tendon and/or nerve transfers are the only option. Steindler flexorplasty is the most commonly used muscle transfer. Nerve transfers include spinal accessory nerve, intercostal nerves and contralateral C7 nerve root. Although not generally accepted, it seems that the overall results of nerve transfer are superior to tendon transfer. In 1994, Oberlin presented a new method for nerve transfer involving transfer of 10% of fascicles [1].

References

1.   Oberlin C, Béal D, Leechavengvongs S, Salon A, Dauge MC, Sarcy JJ. Nerve transfer to biceps muscle using a part of ulnar nerve for C5-C6 avulsion of the brachial plexus: anatomical study and report of four cases. *J Hand Surg [Am]* 1994; 19(2): 232-7.

32 B.

Radialisation involves tendon transfers of radial tendons to create an ulnar balancing force.

33 C.

Is generally not recommended for proximal Urbaniak Class III ring avulsion/amputation injuries. Urbaniak and colleagues classified ring avulsion injuries into Class I (circulation intact), II (compromised circulation requiring revascularisation; no fracture/dislocation) and III (total degloving; may be accompanied by fracture/dislocation); this has since been modified. Ring avulsions with digital amputation have a poor prognosis and are usually better managed by primary amputation, especially if proximal to the FDS tendon insertion. Surviving digital replants exist following 42 hours warm ischaemia and 94 hours cold ischaemia. Especially good outcomes can be achieved with amputations at the level of the DIP joint.

References

1. Urbaniak JR, Evans JP, Bright DS. Microvascular management of ring avulsion injuries. *J Hand Surg [Am]* 1981; 6(1): 25-30.

34 D.

The axillary nerve can be innervated by the nerves to triceps. The intercostal nerves are most commonly used to transfer to the musculocutaneous, thoracodorsal, serratus anterior, pectoral nerves or as donor axons for free muscle transfer. They are very rarely grafted to the median nerve. The phrenic nerve can be used for transfer, particularly if there is an accessory phrenic nerve. The phrenic nerve would not be used if there was a significant chest injury. Transfer of the spinal accessory nerve does not cause loss of function to the trapezius muscle. This is because it can be divided after it has innervated the upper fibres of the trapezius muscle and transferred up, usually to innervate the suprascapular nerve. The axillary nerve can be re-innervated by transferring the nerve to the long head of triceps, which can be sacrificed without undue donor morbidity. This is usually done in combination with an accessory to suprascapular nerve transfer for shoulder function. The contralateral C7 root transfer has been widely used in China and East Asia. This is usually performed in significant avulsion injuries of the contralateral limb. When performed it is usually performed in combination with a vascularised ulnar nerve graft. Complications may include sensory disturbances in the previously intact limb, usually in the index and thumb. Temporary motor deficit is sometimes found with respect to shoulder extension, elbow extension, forearm pronation and wrist extension but full functional recovery is usually documented within 6 months.

35 D.

Glomus tumour. While ganglion cysts and glomus tumours can both cause deformity of the nail plate, the presence of pain and cold sensitivity are highly specific for a glomus tumour. A glomus tumour arises from a glomus body, which functions to regulate peripheral blood flow in response to temperature change. Glomus tumours may involve the nailbed, sometimes causing ridging of the nail plate, and classically present with localised cold intolerance, pain and tenderness. Reproduction of the pain by placing the involved digit into ice-cold water for 1 minute is diagnostic.

References

1.   Shapiro PS, Seitz WH. Non-neoplastic tumors of the hand and upper extremity. *Hand Clin* 1995; 11(2): 133-60.

36 E.

A differential diagnosis includes shoulder injury, cervical cord lesions and arthrogryphosis. The incidence of brachial plexus palsy in the UK is 0.42/1000 live births. This is very similar to the rates described almost 50 years ago, and is despite advances in obstetric care. A possible explanation for this is the increase in birth weight that has been observed over this time. The main associated factors are shoulder dystocia (65%), assisted delivery (ventouse or forceps - 36%), and high birth weight. The incidence of breech delivery in obstetrical brachial plexus palsy is the same as that of the normal population. The most important differential diagnosis is that of shoulder injury. Lack of movement can mimic brachial plexus palsy, but passive range of movement is also affected. Much rarer differentials include cervical cord lesions and arthrogryphosis.

37 B.

Joint mobilisation under anaesthesia. This statement is incorrect; joint mobilisation is not an accepted treatment for arthritis.

38 E.

Multiple slips of both abductor pollicis longus (APL) and extensor pollicis brevis (EPB) can be present. This is incorrect; while multiple slips of APL are common, EPB is normally a single tendon or can be absent in around 5% of cases. Another common anatomical variation is septation of the first dorsal compartment into two distinct tunnels. Finkelstein's test was first described by Eichoff, but was first reported in the American literature by Harry Finkelstein in 1930 [1]. To perform the test, the thumb is placed in a closed fist and the hand is ulnar deviated. If sharp pain occurs along the distal radius, DeQuervain's tenosynovitis is likely.

References
1.   Finkelstein H. Stenosing tendovaginitis at the radial styloid process. *J Bone Joint Surg* 1930; 12: 509-40.

39 E.

Needle fasciotomy is as successful in correcting MCP joint contracture as fasciectomy. However, the recurrence rates are probably higher. Nevertheless, this is balanced by the lower risk of surgery and simplicity of an office procedure, as well as repeatability.

40 B.

Giant cell tumours of tendon sheath recur commonly and are usually benign. Melorheostosis is a rare and progressive disorder characterised by hyperostosis (thickening) of the cortical bone. Melorheostosis affects both bone and soft tissue growth and development. Giant cell tumours of tendon sheath are most likely to recur if disease is left behind and this is more likely where it arises from joints. Despite the high recurrence rate of giant cell tumours, they remain benign in the majority. Acral melanoma occurs on the hand, and is especially common in black skin.

41 A.

Pigmented villonodular synovioma. This is incorrect; pigmented villonodular synovioma usually presents as a non-tender non-inflamed mass.

42 C.

Soucquet-Hoyer. This is incorrect; this is the name of the canals forming the arteriovenous anastomoses. The pin test of Love and the exsanguination test of Hildreth are commonly used tests in the assessment of a potential glomus tumour. Application of cold using ethyl alcohol spray provokes pain and transillumination can show a cherry red mass. Glomus tumours are vascular hamartomas. Although the mechanism of pain generation is uncertain, it is thought to be related to vasodilation and stretch of the Soucquet-Hoyer arteriovenous channels.

43 C.

Liposarcoma. Chondrosarcoma is the most common bone sarcoma seen in the hand and epithelioid sarcoma is the most common soft tissue sarcoma of the hand. Liposarcomata are rarely seen in the hand.

44 D.

Traumatic perforation. Traumatic perforation is not an accepted theory, although microtrauma is considered a potential aetiology, amongst others.

45 E.

Sentinel lymph node biopsy confers staging benefit. This statement is incorrect. Epithelioid sarcoma may be mistaken for other pathology. While SLNB has been described in its management, no unequivocal evidence of benefit has been shown due to a propensity for nodal metastases.

46 B.

Carpal tunnel decompression was first performed in 1896. B is false. Carpal tunnel decompression was probably first performed by Herbert Galloway in 1924. Approximately 20-25% of sufferers are male and approximately 25% of motor branches are transligamental as shown by Lanz. The age of presentation rises towards a peak in the late fifties. Older patients tend to have more severe disease.

47 A.

Ligament of Struthers. This is incorrect; the Ligament of Struthers is an accessory origin for pronator teres and beneath which the median (not ulnar) nerve passes and may be compressed.

48 D.

Can cause Ramsay Hunt syndrome. This is incorrect. Guyon's canal may be divided into three zones, where zone 1 is proximal to the bifurcation of the ulnar nerve into motor and sensory branches and zones 2 and 3 are lie alongside each other. Zone 2 includes the hook of the hamate and surrounds the deep motor branch; zone 3 contains the superficial sensory branch. Ramsay Hunt syndrome (also termed Hunt's syndrome and

Herpes zoster oticus) is a Herpes zoster virus infection of the geniculate ganglion of the facial nerve.

49 E.

Charcot Marie Tooth. In Charcot Marie Tooth, the symptoms are preferentially in the feet and legs and only in the hands later in the disease process. This is classical, and is not a differential.

50 A.

On the right is associated with Poland's syndrome. It is classified as undergrowth in the IFSSH classification, is not confused with constriction ring syndrome, is not treated by pollicisation, and, has short, but not transverse lying bones.

51 B.

Osteoarthritis. These can all be associated with mononeuropathies except osteoarthritis.

52 D.

Bilharzia. Bilharzia is now known as schistosomiasis. Although this can affect many organs (spleen, liver, bowel, kidney, bladder), it can affect the central nervous system but does not affect the peripheral nervous system.

53 C.

Defect in gene for central nerve axonal transport. It is not associated with a defect in the gene for central nerve axonal transport, but rather a defect in the gene for peripheral myelin protein 22 (PMP-22).

54 C.

Avulsion of the lower brachial plexus. At birth, the upper extremity may be flail. Two days following birth, the neurologic examination findings are more reliable. With Erb palsy or upper plexopathy, the arm is internally rotated and pronated with no movement at the shoulder or elbow; hand and wrist flexion are noted. With complete brachial plexus paralysis, the entire arm and hand are flail, with no movement. A Horner syndrome (eyelid ptosis and pupillary miosis) may be noted, suggesting avulsion of the lower brachial plexus. Phrenic nerve palsy suggests a very severe avulsion injury, and urgent plication of the diaphragm may be indicated in patients with pulmonary compromise.

The prognostic value of concurrent Horner's syndrome in infants with total birth palsy was investigated [1]. The records of 48 cases with total palsy were reviewed. Poor spontaneous return of motor function of the limb was found for both with and without concurrent Horner's syndrome. Fisher's exact test (p=0.02) indicated that the presence of concurrent Horner's syndrome is a significant prognostic factor for poor spontaneous recovery of the limb.

References
1.   Al-Qattan MM, Clarke HM, Curtis CG. The prognostic value of concurrent Horner's syndrome in total obstetric brachial plexus injury. *J Hand Surg [Br]* 2000; 25(2): 166-7.

2.   Mackinnon SE. Brachial plexus injuries, obstetrical. eMedicine® from WebMD®.

55 D.

Ectodermal necrosis aetiological theory. D is false. One theory is mesenchymal necrosis.

56 E.

First web space tightness. Thumb hypoplasias are often associated with a narrow/tight first webspace. They are associated with phalangeal and occasionally metacarpal anomalies, but not scaphoid. They are treated according to severity, and in severe cases are treated by pollicisation not toe transfer. Weckesser classified clasped thumb, not hypoplasia.

57 A.

The metacarpal head becomes the new trapezium.

58 C.

Always look for pollex abductus. Pollex abductus is an anomaly in which FPL attaches not only at its customary insertion, but also into the extensor by a tendon that passes around the radial aspect of the thumb. It is of higher incidence in cases of thumb duplication.

59 B.

Pollicisation. In these, there is absence and instability of the proximal thumb metacarpal, and pollicisation is widely recommended.

60 C.

Is associated with autosomal dominant inheritance. Finger nubbins are seen in symbrachydactyly (previously known as atypical cleft hand), not in typical cleft hand. There is no preference for the left hand and usually there is a poor thumb but reasonable function.

61 C.

The median artery can be persistent. The radial structures are hypoplastic and the ulnar soft tissues are not affected.

62 C.

Reconstruction of the ulnar collateral ligament is necessary. This statement is incorrect; reconstruction of the ulnar collateral ligament is unnecessary in most cases of polydactyly which are usually Type A.

63 D.

Muscle and vessel. Although all of the components of a vascularised limb allograft (including skin, subcutaneous tissue, bone, muscle and vessel) are considered highly antigenic, there is a difference between their relative antigenicity. Vascularised muscle allografts can elicit even a stronger cellular response than skin. The least antigenic among these tissues are vessels.

64 E.

Exclusively synovial origins. E is false. Giant cell tumours have been reported in distant sites.

65 D.

A vein graft from the radial artery in the anatomical snuffbox is often necessary. Digital avulsion injuries are accompanied by extended vascular damage with intimal stripping, which require debridement and replacement with good quality vein grafts if replantation is to be successful. Some series quote rates of injuries requiring vein grafts to be in the region of 20%. End-to-side anastomosis of a reversed interpositional vein graft from the radial artery in the snuffbox is one method often used to overcome the vascular gap. The first dorsal metacarpal artery is another useful recipient vessel; this option spares the radial artery in case toe transfer becomes necessary after failed thumb replantation. It is often necessary or desirable to shorten the bone to allow good bony and neurovascular approximation although in the thumb this should be from the amputate and not the residual proximal stump since preservation of length is essential if replantation fails. Repair of FPL should be carried out at the time if possible but secondary reconstruction is sometimes required.

66 B.

The apical ectodermal ridge secretes fibroblast derived growth factor 4.

67 B.

Scapholunate instability. Scapholunate instability is the most common form of carpal instability in terms of anatomical location. It was not until 1972 when Linschied *et al* described the clinical features that this condition became well recognised, although Destot had described the radiological features in 1926. Of the various described carpal instabilities, dorsal intercalated segment instability (DISI) is the most common followed by volar intercalated segment instability (VISI). DISI can be recognised by dorsal tilt of the lunate on a true lateral wrist radiograph associated with volar tilt of the scaphoid, producing a scapholunate angle of greater than 60°. The normal scapholunate angle is 30-60°.

68 B.

Wedge osteotomy of the carpus can improve the hand position.

69 D.

Osteoarthritis of the CMC joint of the thumb. To provide appropriate treatment, DeQuervain's stenosing tenosynovitis needs to be differentiated from intersection syndrome (tendon entrapment of the second extensor compartment) and arthritis of the thumb CMC joint or scaphotrapezial/trapezoid joint.

70 A.

Web creep is less likely to occur if the separation is performed after age two.

71 A.

The A1 pulley alone. In surgical treatment of trigger finger, the A1 pulley is incised - either through an open or a percutaneous approach. It is important to ensure complete release of the annulus that is contributing to the triggering and to avoid injury to the adjacent proximal edge of the A2 pulley. Division of the A1 pulley alone causes no significant loss of flexor function. The oblique pulley in the thumb and A2 pulley in a finger must be preserved when the A1 is divided in order to prevent bowstringing.

72 C.

They occur in 1:150 births. This statement is incorrect; the actual incidence is approximately 1:500 births and are often bilateral. The teratologic sequence of Ogino includes clefting, symbrachydactyly and polydactyly.

73 A.

Intrinsic tightness. A is incorrect. Intrinsic tightness is tested by the Bunnell-Finochietto test. When tightness is present, the PIP joints can be passively flexed without difficulty when the MCP joint is flexed, but are tight when the MCP joint is extended.

74 D.

Thumb surgery is considered a low-risk, high-benefit procedure. Souter from Edinburgh described thumb surgery as a low-risk, high-benefit strategy. He wrote up his extensive series of results from rheumatoid surgeries, and ranked procedures in terms of predictability and efficacy of outcomes.

75 A.

Arthritis of the hand for >6 weeks. To diagnose rheumatoid arthritis, four of the following seven must be present according to the American Academy of Rheumatology: 1) morning stiffness >1hr for >6 weeks; 2) arthritis for >6 weeks in three or more joints; 3) arthritis of the hand for >6 weeks; 4) positive rheumatoid factor; 5) presence of rheumatoid nodules; 6) typical radiographic changes; and, 7) symmetric arthritis for >6 weeks.

76 C.

There is an increased ratio of Type III to Type I collagen. Studies have shown that Dupuytren's aponeurosis collagen has an increased proportion of Type III collagen relative to Type I collagen when compared with age-matched normal aponeurosis tissues.

References

1.   Bailey AJ, Sims TJ, Gabbiani G, Bazin S. Collagen of Dupuytren's disease. *Clin Sci MolMed* 1977; 53 (5): 499-502.
2.   Bazin S, Le Lous M, Duance VC, Sims TJ, Bailey AJ, Gabbiani G, D'Andiran G, Pizzolato G, Browski A, Nicoletis C, Delaunay A. Biochemistry and histology of the connective tissue of Dupuytren's disease lesions. *Eur J Clin Invest* 1980; 10(1): 9-16.
3.   Brickley-Parsons D, Glimcher MJ, Smith RJ, Albin R, Adams JP. Biochemical changes in the collagen of the palmar fascia in patients with Dupuytren's disease. *J Bone Joint Surg [Am]* 1981; 63(5): 787-97.

77 B.

Autosomal dominant. Epidemiological studies on Dupuytren's disease have suggested an inherited mode of transmission that is more commonly autosomal dominant. However, sporadic cases occur and other modes of inheritance have been implicated.

References

1.   Burge P: Genetics of Dupuytren's disease [review]. *Hand Clin* 1999; 15 (1): 63-71.

78 D.

Retrovascular cord of Thomine. The retrovascular cord lies deep (dorsal) to the digital neurovascular bundle. It arises at the proximal phalanx, attaches to the lateral distal phalanx and its development contributes to volar and medial displacement of the neurovascular bundle. It is the usual cause of DIP joint contracture in Dupuytren's disease.

79 E.

None of the above. It is often stated that any contracture of the PIP joint is an indication for surgery, but McGrouther disagrees based on the results of McFarlane and Botz's study which showed that when PIP joint contracture was less than 30°, patients were more often made functionally worse, not better, by surgery. This question highlights this point and the surrounding controversy. MPJ contracture can be corrected no matter how long lasting. As stated by McGrouther, it is most important to show loss of function or progression of disease before submitting the patient to time off work, inconvenience, cost and discomfort without a guaranteed long-term outcome.

References

1.   McGrouther DA. In: *Green's operative hand surgery*, 5th ed. Philadelphia, USA: Elsevier-Churchill Livingstone, 2005: 168.

80 E.

The specificity of nerve conduction studies is less than 70%. This statement is incorrect. The value of nerve conduction studies (NCS) in the diagnosis and evaluation of treatment modalities remains controversial. In 1993, the Quality Assurance Committee of the American Association of Electrodiagnostic Medicine published their critique of the literature available at that time to determine the usefulness of NCS for the evaluation of patients with carpal tunnel syndrome. The specificity of NCS in this circumstance was found to be well in excess of 70% and closer to 95%. The Committee is scheduled to publish a repeat of this study in due course.

References

1.   Jablecki CK, Andary MT, So YT, *et al*. Literature review of the usefulness of nerve
      conduction studies and electromyography for the evaluation of patients with carpal
      tunnel syndrome: AAEM Quality Assurance Committee. *Muscle Nerve* 1994: 17(12):
      1490-1.

81 D.

The Belfast regime is a 'CAM' regime, i.e. controlled active motion. Small
and colleagues, in Belfast, proposed and published their protocol of
controlled early active mobilization of flexor tendons 48 hours following
repair using a Kessler core suture. Its original format has been modified
many times since.

References

1.   Small JO, Brennen MD, Colville J. Early active mobilisation following flexor tendon
      repair in zone 2. *J Hand Surg [Br]* 1989; 14 (4): 383-91.

82 D.

*The ulnar collateral ligament is obstructed by the adductor pollicis
aponeurosis.* The ulnar collateral ligament of the MCP joint of the thumb is
normally covered by the adductor aponeurosis. With marked radial
angulation, the collateral ligament ruptures and the aponeurosis edge
advances distal to the flail end of the ligament. Upon realignment, the
aponeurosis edge sweeps the ulnar collateral ligament proximally and
prevents reapproximation with its distal insertion point. Stener lesions
therefore require surgical reduction and repair.

83 A.

Index - 5° DIP joint, 40° PIP joint, 25° MCP joint. Whilst the most
appropriate angles for individual small joints of the digits is debated in the
literature and are patient-specific, answer A offers the best of the available
choices. The recommended position for the PIP joint varies between

approximately 40 and 55° depending on the finger. The recommended DIP joint position varies between neutral (0°) and 25° by author(s). The MCP joint angle should generally increase from 25° of flexion for the index to 40° for the little.

References

1. Shin AY, Amadio PC. Stiff finger joints. In: *Green's operative hand surgery*, 5th ed. Green DP, Pederson WC, Hotchkiss RN, Wolfe SW, Eds. Philadelphia, USA: Elsevier Churchill Livingstone, 2005: 417-59.

Section 3 questions

Aesthetic surgery

1   Of the following filler substances, which is correctly matched with its trade name?

A.   Hyaluronic acid and Sculptra®.
B.   Hydroxyapatite and Radiesse®.
C.   Acellular cadaveric dermis and Zyderm®.
D.   Large particle hyaluronic acid and Bioalcamid®.
E.   None of the above.

2   Of the following lasers, which is matched with the correct wavelengh?

A. CO_2 and 2940nm.
B.   Erbium-YAG and 10,600nm.
C.   Alexandrite and 755nm.
D.   KTP and 1064nm.
E.   Nd:YAG and 532nm.

3   Select the best answer - the zones of adherence of the lower limb/gluteal area with respect to liposuction are:

A.   Gluteal crease.
B.   Distal iliotibial tract.
C.   Medial middle thigh.
D.   All of the above.
E.   None of the above.

4 The following classifications are relevant to alopecia:

A. Ludwig.
B. Norwood.
C. McCauley.
D. All of the above.
E. None of the above.

5 Which one of the following is false with regards to silicone?

A. Silicone is a polymer of dimethylsiloxane.
B. Short polymer chains form a viscous liquid.
C. Long polymer chains produce solid silicone.
D. It is found in higher concentrations in synthetic infant milk formulae than in the breast milk of augmented patients.
E. None of these is false.

6 Regarding blepharoplasty, which of the following statements about the normal Caucasian eye is incorrect?

A. The lateral canthal angle is normally about 2mm superior to the medial angle giving the eyelids a slightly upward flare.
B. The highest point of the upper lid margin is just medial to the central papillary axis.
C. Typically the eyelid crease measures more in men than women.
D. The lower eyelid rests at the inferior limbus and its lowest point is just lateral to the pupil.
E. The lower lid crease is formed by the insertion of lower eyelid retractors into the skin at this point.

7 Which of the following is not true for a patient seeking lower lid blepharoplasty?

A. A Schirmer I test showing less than 10mm at 5 minutes would be a relative contra-indication.
B. A 'snap' test should always be performed.
C. Excess skin below the level of the orbital margin is usually corrected by lower lid blepharoplasty.
D. Blindness is a rare but recognised complication.
E. Hamra's procedure redistributes the fat rather than excising it.

8 Which of the following techniques of facelift has the highest rate of facial nerve damage?

A. Subcutaneous plane.
B. Deep plane.
C. Minimal access cranial suspension (MACS) lift.
D. Sub-superficial musculo-aponeurotic system (SMAS).
E. Subperiosteal.

9 Which of the following combined procedures is most appropriate?

1. Aggressive midface lift with minimal lower blepharoplasty excision.
2. Aggressive midface lift with aggressive lower blepharoplasty excision.
3. Brow lift first followed by upper blepharoplasty.
4. Upper blepharoplasty first followed by brow lift.

A. 1, 2 and 3 are correct.
B. 1 and 3 are correct.
C. 2 and 4 are correct.
D. 4 only is correct.
E. None is correct.

10 Which of the following techniques of brow lift has the highest rate of skin necrosis?

A.   Subgaleal.
B.   Subperiosteal.
C.   Subcutaneous.
D.   Subepidermal.
E.   None of the above.

11 Which of the following is true of breast implants?

A.   Saline implants have a lower capsular contracture rate than silicone.
B.   Silicone implants have a higher deflation rate than saline.
C.   Textured implants have a higher capsular contracture rate than smooth.
D.   Subglandular placement has a lower capsular contracture rate than submuscular.
E.   None of the above.

12 Theories regarding formation of capsular contracture include:

A.   Biofilm.
B.   Haematoma.
C.   Foreign body reaction mediated through myofibroblasts.
D.   Infection.
E.   All of the above.

13 Botulinum toxin:

A.   Is derived from *Bacillus anthracis*.
B.   Is derived from *Bacillus botulinum*.
C.   May cause hirsutism.
D.   Is derived from spore-forming anaerobic bacteria.
E.   Can cause tetanus.

14 Two hours after blepharoplasty a 60-year-old hypertensive man complains of a swollen, painful right eye and decreased visual acuity. On examination, he has proptosis of the right eye with decreased vision when compared to the left eye. The most appropriate management includes:

A. Head elevation and ice packs.
B. Antihypertensive medication.
C. Diuretics and pain medication.
D. Canthotomy, mannitol and acetazolamide.
E. Consultation with an ophthalmologist.

15 A 45-year-old woman who recently underwent Lasik vision correction is seen in consultation for blepharoplasty. How long following the Lasik procedure would it be appropriate to operate on her?

A. 6 months.
B. 1 month.
C. 18 months.
D. 24 months.
E. 3 months.

16 Three weeks after a facelift, a 56-year-old man suffers an immediate rapidly expanding, painful swelling on the left side of his face while exerting himself. The most likely source of the bleeding is:

A. The external jugular vein.
B. The facial artery.
C. The superficial temporal artery.
D. The facial vein.
E. Generalised subcutaneous oozing.

17 The names of Skoog, Sterzi, Mitz, and Peyronie are associated with:

A. Periosteal flaps for cleft repair.
B. Hypospadias surgery.
C. Breast reduction.
D. Face lifting.
E. Prominent ear correction.

18 The following is true concerning aesthetic subunits of the cheek:

A. There are four overlapping zones.
B. Zone 1 may be divided into three smaller subunits.
C. Zone 4 may be reconstructed with a cervicofacial flap.
D. Reconstruction of zone 1 defects with rhomboid flaps should be superiorly based to avoid trap door effects and minimise postoperative oedema.
E. Anchor sutures to the periosteum along the zygomatic arch and inferolateral orbital rim should not be used to prevent ectropion.

19 Concerning contour defects of the face:

A. Collagen injections only last 3 months or less.
B. Following dermal fat grafts, most of the fat is reabsorbed but 85% of the graft bulk persists.
C. Following autologous fat grafts there is a 25% decline in volume 12 months after injection.
D. Autologous fat should be injected in 5cc aliquots.
E. Suction harvested fat survives better than surgically harvested fat.

20 Which one is true concerning the nose?

A. Is best considered as four discrete 'vaults' based on underlying skeletal structure.

B.   Derives its sensory innervation from the ophthalmic and maxillary divisions of the trigeminal nerve.
C.   Has 10 aesthetic subunits.
D.   Has 11 aesthetic subunits.
E.   Has 12 aesthetic subunits.

21 Anaesthesia of the nasal side wall is best accomplished through infiltration of which one of the following nerves?

A.   Buccal.
B.   Dorsal nasal.
C.   Infra-orbital.
D.   Infratrochlear.
E.   Zygomaticofacial.

22 Which of the following subcutaneous infiltration techniques used in a patient undergoing suction lipectomy has an infiltrate-to-aspirate ratio of 1:1?

A.   Dry.
B.   Superwet.
C.   Tumescent.
D.   Wet.
E.   None of the above.

23 A 40-year-old woman desires improvement of transverse rhytids along the root of the nose. The most appropriate surgical procedure is resection of which of the following muscles?

A.   Corrugator supercilii.
B.   Frontalis.
C.   Orbicularis oculi.
D.   Procerus.
E.   Levator labii superioris alequae nasi.

24 Which of the following anatomic structures of the ear orginates from the second (hyoid) pharyngeal arch?

A.　Antitragus.
B.　Helical root.
C.　Superior helix.
D.　Tragus.
E.　None of the above

25 Concerning the ear:

A.　The superficial temporal artery is the dominant blood supply.
B.　Arnold's nerve supplies the lower lateral portion and inferior cranial surface of the ear.
C.　The tragus, root of the helix and superior helix arise from the first branchial arch and drain to parotid nodes.
D.　The antihelix, antitragus and lobule arise from the third branchial arch and drain to cervical nodes.
E.　The width is approximately 35% of its length.

26 The incidence of prominent ears in the population is estimated to be:

A.　0.2-0.5%.
B.　2-5%.
C.　10-20%.
D.　25-30%.
E.　50%.

27 A 26-year-old woman of Asian descent who underwent rhinoplasty 5 years ago has erosion of the silicone rubber (Silastic) prothesis through the skin of the nasal tip. Physical examination shows a depressed scar in this region. Secondary

rhinoplasty is planned. Use of which of the following grafts for this procedure is most appropriate to minimise volume loss?

A. Dermis + silicone implant.
B. Fat + silicone implant.
C. Muscle.
D. Cartilage.
E. Bone.

28 Which answer is true regarding structural fat grafting?

A. It should never be used in the nose.
B. It can be used to augment midface hypoplasia.
C. It cannot be used for breast augmentation without the Brava® device.
D. There is no risk of blindness when used around the eye, so long as the orbital septum is not breached.
E. HIV is an absolute contraindication.

29 The following are recognised fixation methods for endoscopic brow lift except:

A. Endotine® absorbable devices.
B. Absorbable K-wires.
C. Reconstruction plates.
D. Cortical bone tunnels.
E. Tissue adhesives.

30 Subplatysmal procedures for rejuvenation of the ageing neck include the following except:

A. Open fat excision.
B. Tangential excision of the anterior bellies of digastric.

C.   Intracapsular excision of the superficial portion of the submandibular gland.
D.   Release of the suprahyoid fascia for a high hyoid.
E.   Corset platysmaplasty.

31 The following filler products are matched with various information. When quoted, the estimated number of patients upon which each has been used is correct in all cases. Which one answer is incorrect?

A.   Product: collagen, brand name Zyderm®, persistence 6 months, patients 5 million, granuloma rates (manufacturers) 1:2500.
B.   Product: hyaluronic acid, brand name Restylane®, persistence 12 months, patients 2 million, granuloma rates (manufacturers) 1:50,000.
C.   Product: calcium hydroxyapatite microspheres, brand name Radiesse®, persistence >12 months, granuloma rates (manufacturers) 1:50,000.
D.   Product: polyacrylamide gel, brand name Bioalcamid®, persistence permanent, granuloma rates (manufacturers) 1:5000.
E.   Product: poly-L-Lactic acid, brand name Sculptra®, persistence >12 months, patients 150,000, granuloma rates (manufacturers) 1:500.

32 The following is false about aesthetic breast surgery:

A.   A well-described technique involves positioning of the implant above the pectoralis muscle, but immediately beneath the pectoralis fascia.
B.   Using mesh as an adjunct in mastopexy is well described.
C.   Suction alone for 12 hours a day for 4 weeks can permanently increase the size of breasts, although results are better with autologous fat transfer.

D.   A peri-areolar approach is a poor option through which to adjust the inframammary fold (IMF).
E.   The circumference C of a round breast implant can be calculated using the equation C = 3.14 x the diameter of the implant.

33 Suggested 'ideal' breast measurements in the context of inferior pedicle breast reduction surgery do not include:

A.   Sternal notch to nipple distance of 21cm.
B.   Inter-nipple distance 21cm.
C.   The nipple to inframammary fold distance of 3.4cm.
D.   Areolar diameter 4cm.
E.   A nipple near the mid-humeral point.

34 The following Q-switched laser is least appropriately matched with the pigment colours for which its ablative efficacies are optimal:

A.   Ruby (694) - black, blue and green.
B.   Alexandrite (755) - black, blue and green.
C.   Nd:YAG [KTP] (532) - black, blue and green.
D.   Nd:YAG (1064) - black, blue and green.
E.   All of the above choices are in fact appropriately matched.

35 Which of the following is not a useful nerve block for peri-orbital surgery?

A.   Infra-orbital nerve block.
B.   Zygomaticofacial nerve block.
C.   Frontal nerve block.
D.   Nasociliary nerve block.
E.   Anterior ethmoidal nerve block.

36 The following statement is true with regards to the facial nerve:

A. The buccal branch is crucial for lower eyelid function.
B. The function of the stapedius muscle is lost if the facial nerve nucleus itself is ablated or infarcted, leading to hyperacusis.
C. It is the most commonly damaged nerve during facelift surgery.
D. Branches include the postauricular branch to occipitalis and a branch to the anterior belly of digastric.
E. Damage to the mandibular branch is less likely to cause sequelae than damage to the buccal branch.

37 The following is true in relation to 'malar bags' or festoons:

A. Interestingly, they are hardly ever seen in smokers.
B. They should be excised directly with minimal margins.
C. There is no accepted and routinely successful treatment.
D. They can be treated with minimal-skin-excision lower lid blepharoplasty.
E. They can be significantly improved by a combined course of steroids and diuretics, but only in patients under the age of 40, without comorbidity, and for a maximum period of 4 weeks.

38 The blood vessels immediately supplying the eyelids include all except:

A. Medial superior palpebral artery.
B. Superior arcade.
C. Angular artery.
D. Facial artery.
E. Marginal arcade.

39 Concerning the facial nerves and facelift, which of the following is false?

A.   The frontal branch is found on Pitanguy's line, from 0.5cm below the tragus to 1.5cm above the lateral eyebrow and is accompanied by the anterior branch of the facial artery.

B.   Above the zygoma the nerve runs on the undersurface of the temporoparietal fascia.

C.   McKinney's point refers to the position of the greater auricular nerve, 6.5cm caudal to the external acoustic meatus with the head turned to 45°, at which point it crosses the anterior belly of sternocleidomastoid.

D.   The buccal branch is the most commonly injured branch of the facial nerve during facelift.

E.   If the buccal branch is injured, it is not typically symptomatic as it demonstrates collateral innervation in up to 70% of individuals.

Section 3 answers

Aesthetic surgery

1   B.

Hydroxyapatite and Radiesse®. Hyaluronic acid fillers include Perlane®, Restylane® and Macrolane®. Acellular cadaveric dermis is Alloderm®. Zyderm® is a bovine collagen suspension (as is Zyplast®). Bioalcamid® is a permanent filler consisting of polyalkylamide gel. Sculptra® is poly L-lactic acid.

2   C.

Alexandrite and 755nm. CO_2 is 10,600, ER:YAG is an erbium yttrium aluminium garnet laser at 2940, KTP is potassium titanyl phosphate and is the frequency doubling crystal for Nd:YAG (neodynium YAG), hence halving the Nd:YAG wavelength of 1064 to 532.

3   D.

All of the above. Due attention to liposuction technique around these areas is required to avoid significant contour deformity.

4   D.

All of the above. Ludwig classified into three categories female androgenic alopecia. Norwood classified into seven categories male androgenic alopecia. McCauley classified burn alopecia in the context of feasibility of reconstruction with tissue expansion.

5   C.

Long polymer chains produce solid silicone. C is false. While short polymer chains form a viscous liquid, long chains form a cohesive gel. Solid silicone is formed by cross-linking of the polymer chains. While silicone can be found in the breast milk of implanted patients, it is in lesser quantities than in infant formula milk.

6   C.

Typically the eyelid crease measures more in men than women. This statement is incorrect; the eyelid crease is significantly less in men than women (7-8mm vs 10-12mm), which must be accounted for when planning surgery. The lower lid retractors consist of the capsulopalpebral fascia and the inferior tarsal muscle, and their cutaneous insertion forms the lower lid crease. It is important to know the normal position of the eyelid margins and the eye.

7   C.

Excess skin below the level of the orbital margin is usually corrected by lower lid blepharoplasty. This statement is incorrect. Schirmer's test is for lacrimation. The Schirmer I test is performed without anaesthesia and tests for reflex and basic secretion. Less than 10mm of moistening of the paper at 5 minutes is considered positive. It is worth noting that McKinney and Byun showed that Schirmer's test did not correlate well with post-blepharoplasty dry eyes challenging the rationale for routine use of this test prior to blepharoplasty. Anecdotally, few surgeons actually perform this test routinely. The snap test is for excessive lid laxity and must be assessed prior to surgery. Skin folds below the inferior orbital margin (sometimes called 'festoons') are rarely improved by blepharoplasty alone. Hamra described the redistribution of lower lid fat to restore the contours of youth to the lower lid and avoid the risk of a 'cadaveric' eye.

References

1.	McKinney P, Byun M. The value of tear film breakup and Schirmer's tests in preoperative blepharoplasty evaluation. *Plast Reconstr Surg* 1999; 104(2): 566-9; discussion 570-3.

8 B.

Deep plane. The facial nerve branches travel in the sub-SMAS plane. The deep plane technique requires release of the facial ligaments and resuspension between the branches of the facial nerve and thus carries the highest rate of damage. The subperiosteal plane is at all times deep to the nerve.

9 B.

1 and 3 are correct. Aggressive lower blepharoplasty excision is associated with damage to the structural integrity of the lower lid (and can cause a hollowed out appearance), lower eyelid malposition, dry eyes and/or ectropion. Brow lift may influence the outcome of upper blepharoplasty and thus should be done prior.

10 C.

Subcutaneous. In the subcutaneous technique, skin perforators are divided and skin necrosis is a significant risk.

11 A.

Saline implants have a lower capsular contracture rate than silicone. Capsular contracture rates increase in the presence of foreign material and infection. As such, silicone leak increases rates of contracture (A is true), as does the presence of bacteria (subglandular) (D is false). Whilst silicone implants may rupture, they are unlikely to deflate. Quoted contracture rates are 58% for smooth silicone implants and 8% for textured.

References

1. Coleman, DJ, Foo ITH, Sharpe DT. Textured or smooth implants for breast augmentation? A prospective controlled trial. *Br J Plast Surg* 1991; 44(6): 444-8.

12 E.

All of the above. Each of these has been hypothesised as contributing factors to capsular contracture.

13 D.

Is derived from spore-forming anaerobic bacteria (Clostridium botulinum). Other clostridia include *C. tetani* (tetanus), *C. perfringens* (gas gangrene).

14 D.

Canthotomy, mannitol and acetazolamide. This man has a retrobulbar haematoma which if not treated immediately will lead to blindness. This is a true emergency and if the patient's eyesight is to be saved, immediate and decisive treatment is imperative. There is no time to wait for an ophthalmology consult. Head elevation and ice packs, diuretics and pain medication, and hypertensives are of no immediate value. There is no time to even return to the operating room. Immediate canthotomy to decompress the orbit, with intravenous infusion of acetazolamide and mannitol to reduce intra-ocular pressure, are the emergency treatment. After that, consultation with ophthalmology and all the other options are certainly appropriate. However, for the immediate handling of this acute emergency, D is the only appropriate option.

15 C.

18 months. One of the problems associated with Lasik vision correction surgery is the risk of dry eyes. The procedure affects the protective film over the cornea. It is advisable to wait at least 18 months between such a procedure and a blepharoplasty in order to minimise the risk of postoperative dry eyes.

16 C.

The superficial temporal artery. Most haematomas following a facelift are seen within the first 12-24 hours. These are typically related to an increase in venous pressure as a result of nausea, vomiting, or an increase in blood pressure as a result of anxiety or pain. These early (within 24 hours) haematomas are related to venous bleeding or generalised subcutaneous ooze, very rarely bleeding directly from an arterial vessel. However, a delayed haematoma at 3 weeks is most likely associated with bleeding from the superficial temporal artery. It is therefore advisable that if the superficial temporal artery is encountered during the dissection for the facelift it should be ligated at either end rather than cauterized.

17 D.

Face lifting. Their work on the anatomy of the layers of the facial skin led to the SMAS facelift technique. Skoog headed the unit in Uppsala, Sweden. Peyronie was a French barber, who commanded the surgical corps of Louis XIV.

18 B.

Zone 1 may be divided into three smaller subunits. There are three major aesthetic cheek subunits: the infra-orbital, buccomandibular and pre-auricular subunits. Cheek flaps should be adequately anchored to prevent ectropion of the lower eyelid.

19 B.

Following dermal fat grafts, most of the fat is reabsorbed but 85% of the graft bulk persists.

20 A.

Is best considered as four discrete 'vaults' based on underlying skeletal structure. The nose is best considered as four discrete vaults based on underlying skeletal structure. There are nine aesthetic subunits, these being: the dorsum, two sidewalls, the tip, two alae, two soft triangles, and the columella.

21 C.

Infra-orbital. Anaesthesia of the nasal side wall is best accomplished through infiltration of the infra-orbital nerves, which itself may be undertaken through an intra-oral approach.

References

1.   Moore LK, Dailey AF. Summary of cranial nerves. In: *Clinically oriented anatomy*, 4th ed. Moore LK, Dailey AF, Eds. Philadelphia, USA: Lippincott Williams & Wilkins, 1999: 1082-96.

2.   Zide BM, Swift R. How to block and tackle the face. *Plast Reconstr Surg* 1998; 101(3): 840-51.

22 B.

Superwet. In a patient undergoing suction lipectomy, the superwet subcutaneous infiltration technique has an infiltrate-to-aspirate ratio of 1:1 (Fodor 1986). The tumescent technique has a ration of 2-3ml of infiltrate-to-aspirate (Klein 1987).

References

1.   Klein JA, Pitman, G. Tumescent technique for local anesthesia improves safety in large-volume liposuction. *Plast Reconstr Surg* 1993; 92(6): 1099-100.

2.   Trott SA, Beran SJ, Rohrich RJ, Kenkel J, Adams WP Jr., Klein K. Safety consideration and fluid resuscitation in liposuction: an analysis of 53 consecutive patients. *Plast Reconstr Surg* 1998; 102(6): 2220-9.

23 D.

Procerus. For a 40-year-old woman who desires improvement of transverse rhytids along the root of the nose, procerus resection is the most appropriate surgical procedure.

References
1.   Flowers R, Duval C. Blepharoplasty and periorbital aesthetic surgery. In: *Grabb & Smith's plastic surgery*, 5th ed. Aston SJ, Beasley RW, Thorne CH, Eds. Philadelphia, USA: Lippincott-Raven, 1997: 609.
2.   Knize DM. As anatomically based study of the mechanism of eyebrow ptosis. *Plast Reconstr Surg* 1996; 97(7): 1321-33.
3.   Thorne CH, Aston SJ. Aesthetic surgery of the aging face. In: *Grabb & Smith's plastic surgery*, 5th ed. Aston SJ, Beasley RW, Thorne CH, Eds. Philadelphia, USA: Lippincott-Raven, 1997: 617.

107

24 A.

Antitragus. The antitragus orginates from the middle posterior hillock of the second branchial arch. The other components are formed as follows: the three anterior hillocks of the first arch - the tragus, the crus of the helix, and the helix proper; and the posterior hillocks - the lobule, antitragus and antihelix.

References
1.   Brent B. Reconstruction of auricle: In: *Plastic surgery*. McCarthy JG, Ed. Philadelphia, USA: Saunders, 1990: 2093.

25 C.

The tragus, root of the helix and superior helix arise from the first branchial arch and drain to parotid nodes. The posterior auricular artery is the dominant blood supply of the ear, not the superficial temporal artery.

26 B.

2-5%. The incidence of prominent ears in the population is estimated to be 2-5%.

27 D.

Cartilage. For a 26-year-old woman of Asian descent who underwent rhinoplasty 5 years ago, who has erosion of the silicone rubber (Silastic) prothesis through the skin of the nasal tip and a depressed scar in this region, the use of cartilage grafts for this procedure is most appropriate to minimise volume loss.

References

1.   Karacaoglu E, Kizilkaya E, Cermik H, Zienowicz R. The role of recipient sites in fat-graft survival: experimental study. *Ann Plast Surg* 2005; 55(1): 63-8.

2.   Brenner KA, McConnell MP, Evans GR, Calvert JW. Survival of diced cartilage grafts: an experimental study. *Plast Reconstr Surg* 2006; 117(1): 105-15.

28 B.

It can be used to augment midface hypoplasia. Use of autologous fat in the nose is well described. It can be effective in midface hypoplasia. Although controversial, breast augmentation can be undertaken effectively without pre-expansion with a suction device. The risk of blindness when injecting substances around the eye relates to retrograde propulsion of material along vessels which can occlude the retinal artery, and is limited in its reports to a small number of case reports. HIV lipodystrophy can be treated in this way effectively.

References

1.   Coleman SR, Mazzola RF. *Fat injection: from filling to regeneration.* St. Louis, USA: Quality Medical Publishing Inc., 2009.

29 C.

Reconstruction plates. Fixation methods can be endogenous or exogenous. Although plates have been described for fixation in the endobrow, these are miniplates or resorbable plates. Reconstruction plates are too big and inappropriate for this purpose.

References

1.   Rohrich R, Beran SJ. Evolving fixation methods in endoscopically assisted forehead rejuvenation: controversies and rationale. communications in cosmetic surgery. *Plast Reconstr Surg* 1997; 100(6): 1575-82.

30 E.

Corset platysmaplasty. This is incorrect; corset platysmaplasty is not undertaken deep to platysma, but involves platysma itself. The other listed procedures are well described.

References

1.   Abood A, Malata C. Surgical rejuvenation of the aging neck. In: *The evidence for plastic surgery.* Stone C, Ed. Shrewsbury, UK: tfm publishing Ltd, 2008: 299-310.

31 B.

Product: hyaluronic acid, brand name Restylane®, persistence 12 months, patients 2 million, granuloma rates (manufacturers) 1:50,000. This statement is incorrect; Restylane has a persistence of 6 months not 12, and the quoted manufacturer granuloma rate is 1:2500 not 1:50,000, although published figures from independent authors show granuloma rates of approximately 1:250. A discussion of granulomas should be part of the consent process for any filler injection. The other independent granuloma published rates available for other products are: Zyderm® 1:300, Sculptra® 1:400, Bioalcamid® 1:300. Interestingly, the granuloma rates for permanent silicone gel injections is around 1:1000 (independent and manufacturer's rates).

Reference

1.   Cohen SR, Born TM. Facial rejuvenation with fillers. In: *Techniques in aesthetic surgery*. Codner MA, series editor. Edinburgh: Saunders, 2009.

32 D.

A peri-areolar approach is a poor option through which to adjust the infra-mammary fold (IMF). D is false. The peri-areolar approach allows good access to the IMF. The subfascial position for implants has been reported by both Goes and Graf and may reduce capsular contracture rates. Other positions include the subglandular plane, the subpectoral plane deep to pectoralis major but superficial to minor, a plane beneath both pectoralis and serratus anterior, and the dual plane approach of Tebbetts. Suction as advocated by Khouri and colleagues using the BRAVA® device has purported some success especially with adjunctive fat injection, although the latter technique remains controversial. The circumference of a circle follows the equation 2 x pi x radius (or pi x diameter).

33 C.

The nipple to inframammary fold distance of 3.4cm. C is false. Jack Penn published on the aesthetics of the female breast in 1954 in what was then the *British Journal of Plastic Surgery*. The ideal nipple to IMF distance was quoted as 6.9cm but some think 5-6cm, and it is dependent on technique employed. He stated in the abstract: "it should be within the capacity of plastic surgery to produce a final modelling which should satisfy the strictest artistic criteria". The ideal areolar diameter is approximately 3.8-4.5cm.

34 C.

Nd:YAG [KTP] (532) - black, blue and green. All the Q-switched lasers are effective at removing black pigment, although the frequency doubled Nd:YAG laser (KTP laser) is slightly less efficacious than the others listed. Those lasers in the red or infrared spectrum are more effective at ablating complimentary colours such as green. Hence Alexandrite, Ruby and

Nd:YAG lasers are effective at ablating green and blue pigments. Nd:YAG has less affinity for green and blue pigments compared with KTP and Alexandrite as it is further into the infrared spectrum. However, it is the deepest penetrating laser, and as such can be more efficacious against pigments in deeper layers of the skin. KTP is a green laser and therefore has affinity for red and yellow pigment, with little affinity for blue and green.

References

1.   Dibernardo BE, Pozner JN. Lasers and non-surgical rejuvenation. In: *Techniques in aesthetic surgery.* Codner MA, series editor. Edinburgh: Saunders, 2009.

35 E.

Anterior ethmoidal nerve block. This is not a useful nerve block for peri-orbital surgery. The four major nerve blocks for peri-orbital surgery include the infra-orbital nerve, the zygomaticofacial nerve, the frontal nerve (which anaesthetises the supra-orbital and supratrochlear branches) and the nasociliary block for lacrimal and medial canthal surgery. An isolated anterior ethmoidal block is not undertaken and is included in a nasociliary block.

36 A.

The buccal branch is crucial for lower eyelid function. The medial canthal fibres of the buccal branch of VII are important innervators of the inferior/medial orbicularis. Although innervated by the facial nerve, the cell bodies of origin supplying stapedius lie outside the facial nerve nucleus - hence preserved stapedius function can be of diagnostic use when tested. The most commonly injured nerve during facelift surgery is the greater auricular nerve. Due to greater arborisation, the buccal branch of the facial nerve is less likely to reveal a functional deficit when damaged. Damage to the mandibular branch almost inevitably leads to loss of depressor anguli oris function. The facial nerve supplies the posterior belly of digastric.

37 C.

There is no accepted and routinely successful treatment. Prominence of tissue and skin folds can occur in the malar region with ageing, but in some patients these may present as proliferative skin folds. Lower lid blepharoplasty will not help this condition, which is commoner in smokers. Direct excision is rarely satisfactory and leaves unsightly scars in prominent areas. One approach that can help is subcutaneous dissection and redraping combined with a subperiosteal cheek lift.

References

1.   McCord CD, Codner MA. *Eyelid and periorbital surgery.* St Louis, USA: Quality Medical Publishing Inc., 2008.

38 D.

Facial artery. The facial artery branches into other vessels and eventually supplies the eyelids, including the angular artery. The other vessels or arcades listed directly supply the lids.

References

1.   McCord CD, Codner MA. *Eyelid and periorbital surgery.* St Louis, USA: Quality Medical Publishing Inc., 2008.

39 A.

The frontal branch is found on Pitanguy's line, from 0.5cm below the tragus to 1.5cm above the lateral eyebrow and is accompanied by the anterior branch of the facial artery. A is false. The frontal branch is found on Pitanguy's line, from 0.5cm below the tragus to 1.5cm above the lateral eyebrow and is accompanied by the anterior branch of the temporal artery.

Section 4 questions

Breast, trunk and perineum

1   The following is true regarding vaginal agenesis:

A.   It is caused by a defect in the mesonephric duct.
B.   Urinary abnormailities are rare.
C.   Vascularised bowel is the worst reconstructive option.
D.   Reconstruction should be delayed until an age where intercourse can occur so that reconstructions will remain patent.
E.   Can be treated with a split skin graft.

2   Which of the following arteries does not provide blood supply to the nipple-areola complex (NAC)?

A.   Superior thoracic artery.
B.   Thoraco-acromial artery.
C.   Intercostal perforators.
D.   Internal mammary artery.
E.   Lateral thoracic artery.

3   In 1906, the first myocutaneus flap was described when used to cover a chest wall defect created by a wide mastectomy. His paper was missed until the early 1970s. Who was he?

A.   Verneuil.
B.   Denonvilliers.

C.   Tansini.
D.   Hamilton.
E.   Lillemand.

4   Which of the following nerves provide the main innervation to the NAC?

A.   The 2th lateral intercostal nerve.
B.   The 3th lateral intercostal nerve.
C.   The 4th lateral intercostal nerve.
D.   The 5th lateral intercostal nerve.
E.   The 6th lateral intercostal nerve.

5   Which of the following factors is the most important in choosing a suitable breast reduction technique?

A.   The nipple distance as measured from the suprasternal-notch (SSN).
B.   The nipple distance as measured from the inframammary fold (IMF).
C.   Amount of glandular resection.
D.   BMI and general condition of the patient.
E.   Surgeon's experience.

6   Which statement about the TRAM flap is true?

A.   Fat necrosis is seen in the free flap as commonly as in the pedicled flap.
B.   The free flap is based on the superficial inferior epigastric vessels.
C.   It does not matter if the contralateral or ipsilateral flap is used.
D.   Is more elegant than the DIEP flap.
E.   Is contraindicated in the presence of a Pfannenstiel scar.

4 Breast, trunk and perineum

7 Which of the following MUST be adhered to when undertaking a breast reduction?

A. The new nipple position should always be located at 20-22cm from the suprasternal notch.
B. The nipple should be repositioned at the mid-humeral line.
C. The nipple should be repositioned at 4-5cm from the IMF.
D. The new nipple position is determined by the two-finger manoeuvre at the inframamamry fold (Pitanguy's point) and straying from this position is likely to lead to poor results.
E. None of these options is correct.

8 Which of the following contributes to the blood supply of the breast?

A. Lateral thoracic artery.
B. Second internal mammary artery perforator.
C. Intercostal arteries.
D. Thoraco-acromial artery axis.
E. All of the above.

9 In the hands of an inexperienced plastic surgeon, vertical scar mammaplasty is more predictable except:

A. In breast reduction of less than 500g per side.
B. In breast ptosis with less than 30cm of nipple distance to the SSN.
C. In a patient after massive weight loss (MWL).
D. In a young patient less than 30 years old.
E. In a patient with good skin quality.

10 The most reliable technique of breast reduction to preserve NAC sensitivity is:

A.   The superior pedicle.
B.   The inferior pedicle.
C.   Würinger's septum-based pedicle.
D.   The supermedial pedicle.
E.   The lateral pedicle.

11 Concerning mastopexy:

A.   Ptosis is derived from the Greek word for 'hanging'.
B.   Ptosis is most widely classified with the Rignoew classification.
C.   In grade 2 ptosis the nipple-areola complex is at the IMF but not below.
D.   The Benelli technique does not allow parenchymal repositioning.
E.   Lassus is credited with describing the vertical mastopexy without undermining.

12 With regards to the management of pressure sores, which is true?

A.   Surgical management is preferred.
B.   MRI is a poor modality in the assessment of osteomyelitis.
C.   Serum albumin measurements are helpful as a prelude to surgery.
D.   Herbal remedies +/- acupuncture are often curative.
E.   None of the above.

13 Which of the statements below is not true? Autologous breast reconstruction, compared to implants, provides:

A.   A better sensation of the breast.
B.   An easier oncologic follow-up.
C.   Better control of the breast cancer.

D.   Ultimately a less expensive treatment.
E.   A more aesthetically pleasing and long-lasting result.

14 In the process of breast implant selection, the following are important except:

A.   Soft tissue quality.
B.   Bra and cup size.
C.   Implant volume.
D.   Implant type.
E.   Implant shape.

15 Which of the following statements is incorrect in reference to the dual plane breast augmentation technique?

A.   It has less risk of implant visibility.
B.   It has less risk of implant palpability and sharp transition in the upper pole.
C.   It reduces the double-bubble deformity.
D.   It reduces capsular formation.
E.   The subpectoral dissection is combined with a partial subglandular dissection that extends to a variable distance above the inferior border of the pectoralis major muscle.

16 All statements regarding capsular contracture are correct except:

A.   Using a smooth/saline-filled implant and retropectoral pocket results in greater capsular contracture rates than the retroglandular pocket.
B.   Residual haematoma/seroma may contribute to capsule formation.
C.   Rinsing the pocket with antibacterial solution may reduce the capsular contracture rate.
D.   Polyurethane (PU) implants have reduced capsular contracture rates.
E.   A non-touch technique should provide less bacterial growth with the pocket.

17 Autologous breast reconstruction is not possible with:

A.   A pedicled TRAM flap.
B.   A free TRAM flap.
C.   A pedicled DIEP flap.
D.   A free DIEP flap.
E.   A pedicled latissimus dorsi myocutaneous flap.

18 Which of the following is not true about anatomical implants?

A.   Indicated in patients with minimal soft-tissue coverage.
B.   They may affect the early diagnosis of breast cancer.
C.   They may have a higher rate of rotation.
D.   They can provide better aesthetic outcome.
E.   Require more surgical experience.

19 A 45-year-old woman is scheduled to undergo mastectomy of the right breast followed by reconstruction using a free TRAM flap. She has a 15 pack/year history of cigarette smoking. This patient is at increased risk for development of each of the following postoperative complications except:

A.   Abdominal flap necrosis.
B.   Fat necrosis.
C.   Hernia.
D.   Mastectomy skin flap necrosis.
E.   Lower respiratory infection.

20 Which one of the following statements regarding autologous breast reconstruction is incorrect?

A.   Tissue expanders do not work well for irradiated chest wall breast reconstructions.
B.   The nipple must always be resected in cases of invasive breast cancer at less than 2.5cm of the areola.
C.   Primary reconstruction is usually better than secondary reconstruction.
D.   Skin-sparing mastectomy yields more local recurrences.
E.   Latissimus dorsi is not the ideal flap for large reconstructions.

21 A patient has an isolated right-sided chest wall defect 4cm in diameter involving two ribs with adequate soft tissues. Which reconstruction is the most appropriate treatment?

A.   Nylon or polypropylene mesh only.
B.   Titanium mesh only.
C.   Any mesh with a methylmethacrylate sandwich.
D.   Methylmethacrylate alone or bone graft alone.
E.   None of the above.

22 In relation to penile reconstruction, which one is true?

A.   An ulnar forearm free flap reconstruction has significant advantages over a radial forearm flap reconstruction.
B.   Reconstruction to fulfil sexual function and achieve orgasm is not feasible.
C.   Vascularised bone reconstruction using a free fibular flap is a fallacy.
D.   Penile nerve supply is exclusively from the genitofemoral nerve.
E.   The shaft does not need reconstruction if an adequate glans can be formed.

23 Which of the following statements is true?

A.   A DIEP flap has better perfusion than a free TRAM flap.
B.   A free TRAM flap has a higher fat necrosis rate than a DIEP flap.
C.   In all patients the angiosome of the superficial inferior epigastric artery (SIEA) flap is the same as a DIEP flap.
D.   Abdominal wall morbidity is higher in a DIEP flap than a TRAM flap.
E.   The vascularity of a free DIEP flap is better than a pedicled TRAM flap.

24 Which of the following is not an advantage of immediate breast reconstruction after skin-sparing mastectomy?

A.   Improved cosmesis.
B.   Improved oncologic outcome.
C.   Psychologically beneficial.
D.   Smaller scarring.
E.   None of the above.

25 Which of the following is not an advantage of a free TRAM?

A.   It is better perfused than a pedicled TRAM.
B.   A larger volume of tissue can be reconstructed than a pedicled TRAM.
C.   It has a higher partial flap loss rate in smokers and diabetics.
D.   There is no bulge over the medial IMF.
E.   All of the above.

26 From the following options, which is the least appropriate for reconstruction of a 3cm diameter myelomeningocoele in a 3-month old with spina bifida?

A. Bipedicled flap.
B. Bilateral V to Y advancement flaps.
C. Free anterolateral thigh (ALT) flap.
D. Fasciocutaneous back flap.
E. Rhomboid flap.

27 In terms of breast reduction, which is true?

A. The breasts themselves may increase the body mass index.
B. Hall Findlay uses a superior-lateral pedicle.
C. Lejour's technique includes ultrasound-assisted liposuction.
D. The superior techniques tend to 'bottom out' with time compared with inferior pedicle techniques.
E. None of the above.

28 Good flap options for obliteration of defects of the pleural cavity include all except:

A. Rectus abdominis muscle flap.
B. Serratus anterior muscle flap.
C. Pectoralis major muscle flap.
D. Omentum.
E. Latissimus dorsi myocutaneous flap.

29 A 65-year-old man who underwent three-vessel coronary artery bypass grafting (CABG) 5 weeks ago comes to the office because he has a draining lesion near the sternotomy incision. The CABG procedure included harvest of the patient's left internal mammary artery. Temperature is 38.7°C (101.7°). Physical examination shows a 3mm papule at the manubrium of the healed sternotomy incision. A CT scan of the chest shows a sinus tract leading to the internal sternal plate. In addition to removal of sternal wires and debridement of the wound, which of the following is the most appropriate definitive management?

A. Continuous irrigation.
B. Negative-pressure wound therapy.
C. Omental flap.
D. Right pectoralis major muscle flaps.
E. Left rectus abdominis muscle flaps.

30 In delayed unilateral breast reconstruction with DIEP flaps:

A. The flap should be inset in the position of wherever the mastectomy scar was opened.
B. The flap should be inset inferiorly in the IMF position and the skin between the new IMF and the mastectomy scar should in general be discarded.
C. The flap should be inset inferiorly in the IMF position and the skin between the new IMF and the mastectomy scar should in general not be discarded.
D. The most lateral position of the flap should be well behind the anterior axillary line.
E. The position of the IMF should be mirrored and then cut at the level of the opposite side.

31 The following best classifies a patient with an acute osteomyelitis of the sternum which presents 2 weeks after median sternotomy and coronary grafting, and which is culture positive:

A.   Pairolero Type A.
B.   Pairolero Type B.
C.   Pairolero Type C.
D.   All of the above.
E.   None of the above.

32 Which one of the following statements regarding Poland's syndrome is false?

A.   It was first described by Alfred Poland in 1841.
B.   It is more common in men.
C.   A pedicled latissimus flap is suitable for reconstruction of the anterior axillary fold.
D.   A wide range of deformities of the breasts, thoracic wall, pectoralis major, upper limbs and hands is possible.
E.   Its incidence is 1:2500 live births.

33 The following is false in breast reconstruction:

A.   TRAM flaps reduce abdominal wall strength compared with DIEP flaps with resultant detriment to activities of daily living and quality of life.
B.   Pedicled TRAM flaps result in greater morbidity than DIEP flaps from partial flap loss and fat necrosis.
C.   DIEP flaps are associated with reduced immediate/early postoperative pain compared with TRAM flaps.
D.   There is no evidence that shows an increase in abdominal hernias with TRAM flaps compared with DIEP flaps.
E.   TRAM flaps produce comparable aesthetic breast reconstructions and comparable patient satisfaction.

34 The following statements are true except:

A. Cutaneous perforators that do not originate from the deep inferior epigastric artery (peritoneocutaneous perforators) are rare findings when raising a DIEP flap.

B. Pre-operative evaluation of the vasculature of the abdominal wall has been shown to reduce operating times in perforator flap reconstruction.

C. The use of computed tomography of the abdominal wall has been shown to be cost-effective in some studies.

D. The radiation exposure associated with computed tomographic angiography of the abdominal wall is similar to a background radiation dose of 2.5 years.

E. The use of the DIEP flap to reconstruct lower limb defects has not been described.

Section 4 answers

Breast, trunk and perineum

1 E.

Can be treated with a split skin graft. McIndoe's technique of a reversed split skin graft over a stent was presented as a Hunterian Oration in the 1940s. It requires persistent stent usage, and often contracts, but can result in an acceptable reconstruction. Urinary abnormalities are commonly found in vaginal agenesis (Mayer-Rokitansky-Kuster-Hauser syndrome), and should be excluded. Vascularised bowel is a reasonable option, although they can bleed and secrete excessive mucus. Early reconstruction is preferred before sexual awareness of the child, minimising psychological trauma. The defect is of the paramesonephric duct (Mullerian duct).

2 A.

Superior thoracic artery. The superior thoracic artery does not nourish the NAC. The main blood supply to the nipple-areola complex is provided by branches from the internal mammary and the lateral thoracic arteries, which run in the subcutaneous tissue and communicate with each other above and below the areola. The dermal and subdermal vascular plexus has less importance in NAC blood supply. A medial or lateral pedicle provides the best blood supply to the NAC intercostal perforators and the branches from thoraco-acromial artery also contribute to the blood supply of breast tissue. Branches from the thoracodorsal artery may supply the lateral part of the breast.

References

1.	Nakajima H, Imanishi N, Aiso S. Arterial anatomy of the nipple-areola complex. *Plast Reconstr Surg* 1995; 96(4): 843-4.

2.	Hamdi M, Wuringer E, Schlenz I, Kuzbari R. Anatomy of the breast: a clinical application. In: *Vertical scar mammaplasty.* Hamdi M, Hammond DC, Nahai F, Eds. Berlin, Germany: Springer-Verlag, 2005: 1-10.

3   C.

Tansini. Tansini described the latissimus dorsi flap which he undertook in 1897 and published in 1906.

References

1.	Tansini I. Sopra il mio nuovo processo di amputazione della mamella. *Riforma Med* 1906; 12: 757 and *Gazetta Medica Italiana* 1906; 57: 141.

2.	Hutchins EH. A method for the prevention of elephantiasis. *Surg Gynec Obst* 1939; 69: 795.

3.	Campbell DA. Reconstruction of the anterior thoracic wall. *J Thoracic Surg* 1950; 19(3): 456-61.

4   C.

The 4th lateral intercostal nerve. The breast is innervated by lateral and anterior cutaneous branches of the second to the sixth intercostal nerves. The NAC is always innervated by both the anterior and lateral 3th-5th intercostal nerves. The deep branches of the lateral nerves run below or within the pectoralis fascia. At the mid-clavicular line, they turn 90° and continue through the glandular tissue towards the posterior surface of the nipple. The 4th lateral cutaneous branch is the most constant nerve to the nipple, observed in 93% of breasts. The anterior cutaneous branches of the intercostal nerves travel superficially to reach the medial edge of the areola.

References

1.	Schlenz I, Kuzbari R, Gruber H, Holle J. The sensitivity of the nipple-areola complex: an anatomic study. *Plast Reconstr Surg* 2000; 105(3): 905-9.

5   E.

Surgeon's experience. Several techniques in breast reduction are available. Choosing the appropriate procedure depends on many factors. The amount of breast resection, which is obviously related to breast size, is considered one of the most important factors. However, training of the surgeon in a specific technique may make it suitable for use on any breast size. Degree of ptosis and the distance of the nipple to the IMF will determine the length of the pedicle which is needed to carry the NAC. Master plastic surgeons may be able to produce safe techniques in breast reduction; however, free nipple techniques should be considered in inexperienced hands in situations such as elderly patients in poor medical health or with resections more than 2500g per side. There is no best method of breast reduction. The ideal technique may be the one which the surgeon has mastered with the most confidence.

6   E.

Is contraindicated in the presence of a Pfannenstiel scar.

References

1.   Hamdi M, Hall-Findlay EJ. Pedicle choices in breast reduction. In: *Vertical scar mammaplasty*. Hamdi M, Hammond DC, Nahai F, Eds. Berlin, Germany: Springer-Verlag, 2005: 11-6.

7   E.

None of these options is correct. Most aesthetic measurements of the breast are based on Penn's publication which are only a guide. In a group of 20 women with aesthetically perfect breasts, he found the ideal position of the nipple is located at 21cm from the SSN. Mid-humeral measurement was popularised by Lassus. Locating the new nipple position at 4-5cm higher than the IMF is used in inverted-T mammaplasty and does not apply to all techniques. Pitanguy put the nipple where one index in the IMF touches the other index crossing the breast parenchyma. All these measurements can be used as a good starting point; however, more variations have been demonstrated by many other surgeons. Surgeons need to drop the nipple position at least 2cm from their usual design with the inverted-T approach. Vertical mammaplasty creates a significant breast projection and the nipple will have the illusion of being higher because of the increased slope of the upper portion of the breast. Therefore, the new nipple position needs to be lowered about 2cm below what one would use to mark in the inverted-T approach.

References

1.   Penn J. Breast reduction. *Br J Plast Surg* 1955; 7: 357.
2.   Hall-Findlay EJ, A simplified vertical reduction mammaplasty: shortening the learning curve. *Plast Reconstr Surg* 1999; 104(3): 748-59.

8   E.

All of the above.

9   C.

In a patient after massive weight loss (MWL). The ideal candidate for vertical scar mammaplasty is one who has simple breast ptosis or who requires gland reduction of 400-500g or less. A patient of stable weight is preferable to an obese patient whose weight is constantly fluctuating. Young patients usually have good quality skin. Juvenile patients are more prone to unpredictable and hypertrophic scars. The vertical scar often has the least risk as compared with the peri-areolar and the horizontal scars, but all efforts should be undertaken to keep scars as short as possible. Patients with large breasts, where the amount of tissue resection exceeds 1000g per side, and older patients, where skin has lost its elasticity, are not good candidates for this technique. Patients after massive weight loss are better managed with an inverted-T scar technique. Using vertical scar mammaplasty will lead to early ptosis, residual skin excess, and lack of projection of the breast due to flaccid and loose tissue.

References

1.   Hamdi M, Hall-Findlay EJ. Pedicle choices in breast reduction. In: *Vertical scar mammaplasty.* Hamdi M, Hammond DC, Nahai F, Eds. Berlin, Germany: Springer-Verlag, 2004.

10 c.

Würinger's septum-based pedicle. Using a central pedicle or laterally based inferior pedicle technique resulted in loss of nipple sensitivity in 9.5% of breasts and correlated with increasing breast size and amount of resection. When <440g per breast was resected, nipple sensation was retained 100% of the time. Loss of sensation to the nipple can occur after any kind of breast reduction, but some subgroups of patients and reduction techniques are associated with a higher incidence of nipple sensitivity loss than others. Inferior pedicle techniques retain NAC sensitivity better than the superior pedicle techniques during the first 3 months postoperatively. At 6 months postoperatively NAC sensation was comparable between the two techniques. Medial pedicle techniques seem to retain similar NAC sensation as compared with the inferior pedicle technique. Mammaplasty techniques which are based on Würinger's septum seem to preserve sensation to the NAC better. This is a ligamentous suspension of the breast consisting of a horizontal septum attaching the NAC to the thoracic wall at the level of the fifth rib. It also includes branches and perforators from the intercostal, thoraco-acromial, and lateral thoracic vessels as well as the deep branch of the 4th intercostal nerve. Including the septum in a lateral pedicle technique will provide better NAC sensitivity than a traditional superior or inferior pedicle technique.

129

References

1.   Gonzalez F, Brown FE, Gold ME, Walton RL, Shafer B. Preoperative and postoperative nipple-areola sensibility in patients undergoing reduction mammaplasty. *Plast Reconstr Surg* 1993; 92(5): 809-14.

2.   Hamdi M, Greuse M, DeMey A, Webster MHC. A prospective quantitative comparison of breast sensation after superior and inferior pedicle mammaplasty. *Br J Plast Surg* 2001; 54(1): 39-42.

3.   Nahabedian MY, Mofid MM. Viability and sensation of the nipple-areola complex after reduction mammaplasty. *Ann Plast Surg* 2002; 49(1): 24-31.

4.   Würinger E, Mader N, Posch E, Holle J. Nerve and vessel supplying ligamentous suspension of the mammary gland. *Plast Reconstr Surg* 1998; 101(6): 1486-93.

5.   Hamdi M, Blondeel P, Van de Sijpe K, Van Landuyt K, Monstrey S. Evaluation of nipple-areola complex sensitivity after the latero-central glandular pedicle technique in breast reduction. *Br J Plast Surg* 2003; 56(4): 360-4.

11 E.

Lassus is credited with describing the vertical mastopexy without undermining. Regnault classified ptosis in terms of the nipple position in relation to the IMF. The etymology of ptosis is from the Greek 'to fall, falling'.

12 C.

Serum albumin measurements are helpful as a prelude to surgery. Albumin is one serological marker of nutritional status. It is imperative that patients are nutritionally optimised prior to any surgery. Surgical treatment is only undertaken for the minority of pressure sores. MRI is one of the best investigations for osteomyelitis with high sensitivity and specificity.

References

1. Huang AB, Schweitzer ME, Hume E, Batte WG. Osteomyelitis of the pelvis/hips in paralyzed patients: accuracy and clinical utility of MRI. *J Comp Assist Tomogr* 1998; 22(3): 437-43.

13 C.

Better control of the breast cancer. C is false.

14 B.

Bra and cup size. Bra and cup sizes are highly variable among manufacturers and even among countries. In addition, patient understanding of breast size as related to cup size is inaccurate. Several methods have been suggested to predict the appropriate size of an implant for breast augmentation. The pre-operative decision-making process is extremely important for the aesthetic outcome. Many factors should be considered in order to choose a suitable implant. Long-term outcome results depend on the quality of the envelope, implant characteristics, and the surgical technique. Tebbetts and Adams recommend the following implant assessment, referred to as "the high five critical decisions":

1. Optimal soft tissue coverage (pocket location).
2. Implant volume (weight).
3. Implant type and dimensions.
4. Position of the IMF.
5. Incision location.

With this process, the authors reported a 2.8-3% re-operation rate in 2000 patients followed up for more than 6 years.

References

1.   Tebbetts JB, Adams WP. Five critical decisions in breast augmentation using five measurements in five minutes: the high five decision support process. *Plast Reconstr Surg* 2005; 116(7): 2005-16.

15 D.

It reduces capsular formation. This statement is incorrect. Dual plane augmentation is mainly indicated when soft tissue coverage is inadequate. It is a versatile technique because the extent of the subglandular dissection can be tailored to the degree of breast ptosis and allows for implant placement partially under the pectoralis major muscle. The soft tissue is redraped over the lower aspect of the implant. By this, the dual approach combines the advantages of both retropectoral and retroglandular approaches. Although retropectoral approaches report less capsular formation than retroglandular approaches, capsule formation is not solely related to the location of the pocket.

References

1.   Tebbetts JB. Dual plane breast augmentation: optimizing implant-soft-tissue relationships in wide range of breast types. *Plast Reconstr Surg* 2001; 107(5):1255-72.

16 A.

Using a smooth/saline-filled implant and retropectoral pocket results in greater capsular contracture rates than the retroglandular pocket. This statement is incorrect; the aetiology of capsular contracture is still not clear. However, there are two hypotheses: hypertrophic scar formation (haematoma, granulomas, hereditary diseases, etc.) and infection. Myofibroblasts are known to be present on the capsule around the implants. They contribute to capsular contracture as part of the foreign body reaction initiated by silicone. Subclinical infections have also been implicated as a major contributor to capsular contracture. *Staphylococcus epidermidis* was the dominant organism found among culture specimens taken from open capsulectomies. *S. epidermidis* seems to correlate strongly with capsular contracture incidence. The no-touch technique using a sterile sheath to introduce the implant without contact with the skin should provide less capsular contracture. Using preventive antibiotic irrigation of the pocket is also effective. Capsular contracture is less reported with saline implants, low-bleed silicone implants, textured implants, submuscular placement, and in primary augmentation. Polyurethane-covered implants were reported to have the least capsular formation, but they have been banned in the USA since the eighties due to sarcoma induction risk demonstrated in mice. This risk has not been proved in humans and PU implants have been used widely in South America and in some European countries.

References

1.   Prantl L, Schreml S, Fichtner-Feigl S, Poppl N, Eisenmann-Klein M, Schwarze H, Fuchtmeier B. Clinical and morphological conditions in capsular contracture formed around silicone breast implants. *Plast Reconstr Surg* 2007; 120(1): 275-84.

2.   Dobke MK, Svahn JK, Vastine VL, Landon BN, Stein PC, Parsons CL. Characterization of microbial presence at the surface of silicone mammary implants. *Ann Plast Surg* 1995; 34(6): 563-71.

3.   Mladick RA. No-touch submuscular breast augmentation technique. *Aesth Plast Surg* 1993; 17(3): 183-92.

4.   Adams WP Jr, Rios JL, Smith S. Enhancing patient outcomes in aesthetic and reconstructive breast surgery using triple antibiotic breast irrigation: six-year prospective clinical study. *Plast Reconstr Surg* 2006; 117(1): 30-6.

5.   Hester TR, Tebbetts JB, Maxwell GP. The polyurethane-covered mammary prosthesis: facts and fiction (II): a look back and a 'peek' ahead. *Clin Plast Surg* 2001; 28(3): 579-86.

17 C.

A pedicled DIEP flap.

18 B.

They may affect the early diagnosis of breast cancer. This statement is incorrect. The development of anatomical implants added more options to breast augmentation. Using anatomical implants has the following advantages: decreases tendency of upper-pole fullness, edge visibility and roundness, allows more natural breast projection, and gives better volume support for the lower pole of the breast. Due to the risk of rotation, careful implant selection and a 'just-adequate' pocket is essential to avoid this complication, which is estimated at a 1-2% rate. Therefore, using anatomical implants requires more clinical experience. Most anatomical implants are newly developed and use the less-bleeding cohesive-gel silicone, which improves implant safety and reduces capsular contracture. For all these reasons, favourable aesthetic results are reported with anatomical implants. Several studies have shown that breast implants, whatever the kind, do not affect the early diagnosis of breast cancer or the stage at diagnosis.

References

1.   Heden P, Bone B, Murphy DK, Slicton A, Walker PS. Style 410 cohesive silicone breast implants: safety and effectiveness at 5 to 9 years after implantation. *Plast Reconstr Surg* 2006; 118(6): 1281-7.

19 B.

Fat necrosis.

References

1.   Chang DW, Reece GP, Wang B, Robb G, Miller MJ, Evans, GR, Langstein HN, Kroll, SS. Effect of smoking on complications in patients undergoing free TRAM flap breast reconstruction. *Plast Reconstr Surg* 2000; 105(7): 2374-80.
2.   Chang LD, Bunke G, Slezak S. Cigarette smoking, plastic surgery, and microsurgery. *J Reconstr Microsurg* 1996; 12(7): 467-74.

3. Reus WF, Robinson MC, Zachary L. Acute effects of tobacco smoking on blood flow in the cutaneous micro-circulation. *Br J Plast Surg* 1984; 37(2): 213-4.
4. Van Adrichmen LN, Hoegen R, Hovious SE, Kort WJ, van Strik RD, Vuzevski VD, van der Meulen JC. The effect of cigarette smoking on the survival of free vascularized and pedicled epigastric flaps in the rat. *Plast Reconstr Surg* 1996; 97(1): 86-96.

20 D.

Skin-sparing mastectomy yields more local recurrences. This statement is incorrect; breast reconstruction with autologous tissue has no interference on local recurrences.

21 E.

None of the above. None of these options is appropriate. In general, chest wall reconstruction is only indicated in large defects where more than four ribs are missing.

22 A.

An ulnar forearm free flap reconstruction has significant advantages over a radial forearm flap reconstruction. The ulnar forearm flap provides a longer pedicle than the radial flap, good sensation, and most importantly the urethra is cited along a less hair-bearing area of the flap (Lovie 1984, popularised by Gilbert 1995). Pudendal nerve to antebrachial nerve anastomoses can provide good sensory recovery. Vascularised bone flaps have been described. Penile nerve supply is from the pudendal, ilio-inguinal and genitofemoral nerves.

References
1. Mathes SJ, Hentz VR. *Plastic surgery.* St. Louis, USA: Saunders-Elsevier, 2006.

23 E.

The vascularity of a free DIEP flap is better than a pedicled TRAM flap. The DIEP flap is based on one or several perforators that directly fill some of

4 Breast, trunk and perineum

the ipsilateral zone 1, and flow though adjacent choke zones to the adjacent abdominal wall zones. The free TRAM captures this zone 1 territory more completely by including all perforators (A and B are false). The pedicled TRAM is based on the deep superior epigastric artery and thus flow is across a choke zone to reach zone 1, and two major choke zones to reach zones 2 and 3 (E is true). The SIEA angiosome is different to the DIEA angiosome. The DIEP flap spares rectus muscle fibres, unlike the TRAM flap.

24 B.

Improved oncologic outcome. There is no diminished oncologic outcome in selected immediate breast reconstruction; however, there is no actual benefit.

25 C.

It has a higher partial flap loss rate in smokers and diabetics. Options A, B and D are all advantages of the free TRAM over the pedicled TRAM. Option C is true of a pedicled TRAM - a free TRAM has a lower partial flap loss rate.

26 C.

Free anterolateral thigh (ALT) flap. A free flap is not indicated here and is especially challenging in such a young child. Local flaps as described are effective with minimal donor morbidity.

27 A.

The breasts themselves may increase the body mass index. In the context of both abdominoplasty and breast reduction, the tissue requiring resection can itself contribute to the BMI in a minority of cases [1]. Hall Findlay uses a superomedial pedicle. Lejour's original description included standard liposuction and undermining, differentiating from Claude

Lassus's technique. However, further papers by Lejour showed modification of the technique to reduce the relatively high complication rates by minimising undermining and hence revisiting the concepts of Lassus. It is the inferior pedicle technique that has been criticised most for 'bottoming out'.

References

1. Dafydd H, Juma A, Meyers P, Shokrollahi K. The contribution of breast and abdominal pannus weight to body mass index: implications for rationing of reduction mammaplasty and abdominoplasty. *Ann Plast Surg* 2009; 62(3): 244-5.

28 E.

Latissimus dorsi myocutaneous flap. Latissimus dorsi is a useful flap for reconstruction of pleural defects as a muscle flap but not as a myocutaneous flap. The other flaps listed all have indications in this role.

29 D.

Right pectoralis major muscle flaps.

References

1. Ascherman JA, Patel SM, Malhotra SM, Sameer M, Smith CR. Management of sternal wounds with bilateral pectoralis major myocutaneous advancement flaps in 114 consecutively treated patients: refinements in techniques and outcomes analysis. *Plast Reconstr Surg* 2004; 114(3): 676-83.
2. Pairolero PC, Arnold PG. Management of infected median sternotomy wounds. *Ann Thorac Surg* 1986; 42 (1): 1-2.
3. Pairolero PC, Arnold PG, Harris JB. Long term results of pectoralis major muscle transposition for infected sternotomy wounds. *Ann Surg* 1991; 213(6): 583-90.
4. Gur E, Stern D, Weiss J, Herman O, Wertheym E, Cohen M, Shafir R. Clinical-radiological evaluation of poststernotomy wound infection. *Plast Reconstr Surg* 1998; 101(2): 348-55.

30 B.

The flap should be inset inferiorly in the IMF position and the skin between the new IMF and the mastectomy scar should in general be discarded. In delayed unilateral breast reconstruction with DIEP flaps, the aesthetic units of the breast should be taken into consideration. This means that the IMF and lateral border marked by the anterior axillary line should be kept in mind. The lateral part should stop at the anterior axillary line. The IMF should be mirrored to the opposite side but then cut to be 2cm higher as that side will come down slightly more than the unaffected side. All skin between the old mastectomy scar and the new IMF should be discarded to give the best aesthetic result.

31 B.

Pairolero Type B. Pairolero classified sternal osteomyelitis into three categories. The first is characterised by a culture-negative serous discharge within days of surgery without cellulitis, chondritis or osteomyelitis. The second is acute, suppurative and culture positive osteomyelitis, and the third presents months after surgery and is often an acute-on-chronic osteomyelitis.

32 E.

Its incidence is 1:2500 live births. E is false. Poland's syndrome is a rare congenital anomaly characterised by unilateral chest wall hypoplasia and ipsilateral hand abnormalities. Literary data suggest its sporadic nature. The prevailing theory of its cause is hypoplasia of the subclavian artery or its branches, which may lead to a range of developmental changes. The incidence of Poland's syndrome varies between groups (e.g. male versus female patients, congenital versus familial cases) and ranges from 1 in 7,000 to 1 in 100,000 live births.

References

1.   Fokin AA, Robicsek F. Poland's syndrome revisited. *Ann Thorac Surg* 2002; 74(6): 2218-25.

33 A.

TRAM flaps reduce abdominal wall strength compared with DIEP flaps with resultant detriment to activities of daily living and quality of life. A is false. There is no evidence that the preservation of abdominal wall strength from DIEP flaps versus TRAM flaps translates to better maintenance of activities of daily living. Pedicled TRAM flaps are purported to have a higher incidence of flap necrosis and partial flap loss compared with free flaps. DIEP flaps are associated with less postoperative pain than TRAM flaps. There is no evidence than TRAM flaps result in abdominal hernias compared with DIEP flaps.

34 E.

The use of the DIEP flap to reconstruct lower limb defects has not been described. This statement is incorrect; the use of DIEP flaps to reconstruct lower limb defects in 25 patients with promising results was described in 2005 [1]. A study of 375 DIEA perforator (DIEP) flaps (325 with pre-operative CTA and 50 cadaveric dissections) showed that peritoneal-cutaneous perforators were rare anatomical variations (4/375: 1.1%) and that they may affect outcomes in DIEP flap surgery if not assessed pre-operatively. Computed axial tomography (CTA) was significantly able to detect this anomaly and aid operative planning [2]. In a study of 138 DIEP breast reconstructions, 70 underwent pre-operative CTA analysis, and 68 had pre-operative Doppler investigation. Surgery time in the CTA group was significantly lower ($p<0.001$) than in the control group (264min [SD+/-62] versus 354min [SD+/-83]), respectively. The study suggested that the use of CTA helped reduce surgery time, and reduce the risk of postoperative complications [3]. In addition, the time saved during DIEP flap surgery was shown to compare favourably to the cost of the computed tomographic angiography pre-operatively [4]. A paper reviewing the radiation dose of routine investigations compared it to abdominal wall CTA and the background equivalent radiation dose (Table 1) [5].

Table 1. Radiation exposure with CTA in DIEP flap planning.

Investigation	Effective dose	Background equivalent radiation dose
Chest X-ray	0.02mSv	3 days
Abdominal X-ray	0.5mSv	2.5 months
Head CT	2mSv	10 months
Cervical spine CT	3mSv	15 months
Chest CT	5mSv	2 years
Abdo-pelvis CT	10mSv	4 years
Full trauma CT	25mSv	10 years
Abdominal wall CTA	6mSv	2.5 years

Exposure calculated with ImPACT CT Patient Dosimetry Calculator (Version 0.99w, ImPACT, St. George's Hospital, London, UK). Equivalent background radiation dose calculated based on background of 2.42mSv/year.

References

1   Van Landuyt K, Blondeel P, Hamdi M, Tonnard P, Verpaele A, Monstrey S. The versatile DIEP flap: its use in lower extremity reconstruction. *Br J Plast Surg* 2005; 58(1): 2-13.

2.   Whitaker IS, Rozen WM, Smit JM, Dimopoulou A, Ashton MW, Acosta R. Peritoneo-cutaneous perforators in deep inferior epigastric perforator flaps: a cadaveric dissection and computed tomographic angiography study. *Microsurgery* 2009; 29(2): 124-7.

3.   Smit JM, Dimopoulou A, Liss AG, Zeebregts CJ, Kildal M, Whitaker IS, Magnusson A, Acosta R. Preoperative CT angiography reduces surgery time in perforator flap reconstruction. *J Plast Reconstr Aesthet Surg* 2008, Jul 31.

4.   Rozen WM, Ashton MW, Whitaker IS, Wagstaff MJ, Acosta R. The financial implications of computed tomographic angiography in DIEP flap surgery: a cost analysis. *Microsurgery* 2009; 29(2): 168-9.

5.   Rozen WM, Whitaker IS, Stella DL, Phillips TJ, Einsiedel PF, Acosta R, Ashton MW. The radiation exposure of computed tomographic angiography (CTA) in DIEP flap planning: low dose but high impact. *J Plast Reconstr Aesthet Surg* 2008, Dec 31.

Section 5 questions

Burns and trauma

1   When considering the topic of reconstructive burn surgery, which of the following statements do you consider to represent the greatest consensus view?

A.   Reconstructive burns surgery should begin when all scars are fully mature.

B.   In children reconstructive burn surgery should be delayed until puberty.

C.   Reconstructive burn surgery is primarily involved with the release of contractures.

D.   Reconstructive burn surgery should begin in the acute burn phase.

E.   The principal goal of reconstructive burns surgery is independent mobility.

2   Systemic effects of a major burn include:

A.   Increased venous return.

B.   Increasing cardiac preload.

C.   Decreased systemic vascular resistance.

D.   Increased pulmonary vascular resistance.

E.   Hyperproteinaemia.

3 When considering burn reconstruction of the head and neck where the eyes, nose, mouth, ears and scalp are all significantly involved what would be the usual order for priority of reconstruction?

A.   Eyes, ears, nose, mouth, scalp.
B.   Nose, eyes, mouth, scalp, ears.
C.   Mouth, eyes, nose, ears, scalp.
D.   Eyes, mouth, scalp, nose, ears.
E.   Eyes, scalp, mouth, ears, nose.

4 Regarding Integra®, which of the following statements is true?

A.   A major drawback in the use in burns reconstruction is that Integra® contracts.
B.   Integra® is a biodegradable skin regeneration template.
C.   Integra® contains cross-linked Type I bovine tendon collagen and a shark-derived glycosaminoglycan (chondroitin-4-sulphate).
D.   Integra® is microbiologically inert and easily causes infection.
E.   Integra® is a bilaminar biodegradable tissue engineered dermal matrix generation template.

5 There are few published series of microsurgical reconstruction in post-burn paediatric patients. What is the principal reason for this?

A.   Microvascular anastomosis has an unacceptably high failure rate after thermal injury in children.
B.   Children with extensive post-burn contractures do not tolerate prolonged anaesthesia well.
C.   The technical skills to perform these procedures are extremely demanding.

D.   Where the technical skills and resources exist there are relatively few patients who can benefit from the surgery.
E.   Acute burns care is so good that, globally, there is little need for such complex surgery.

6 The following is true regarding fasciotomies of the foot:

A.   The medial approach is a single incision, and provides access to all three compartments.
B.   The lateral approach is the most commonly used.
C.   The dorsal approach is a single incision.
D.   The dorsal approach involves four incisions.
E.   None of the above.

7 Calorific requirements for burn-injured adult patients are:

A.   Calculated based on the Cuschieri formula.
B.   Ideally adjusted for a calorie-nitrogen ratio of 500:1.
C.   25kcal/kg + 40kcal/% burn.
D.   20kcal/kg in children.
E.   Must be given parenterally whenever possible.

8 When looking at the successful outcome of post-burn surgical functional reconstruction which of the following do you think is the most critical determinant of the final result?

A.   The expertise and experience of the reconstructive burns surgeon.
B.   The socio-economic status of the patient.
C.   The expertise and experience of the postoperative rehabilitation therapists.
D.   The motivation and compliance of the patient (and/or parents).
E.   The provision of state-of-the-art equipment for both inpatient and outpatient postoperative physiotherapy and occupational therapy.

9   When considering the aesthetic reconstruction of post-burn facial scarring which has resulted in extensive textural abnormality but no deformity of anatomical features, which of the following would be your method of choice for skin resurfacing?

A. Full thickness excision in anatomic units and grafting with thick split thickness grafts using multiple quilting sutures.

B. Full thickness excision in anatomical units and grafting with pre-expanded full thickness skin.

C. Full thickness excision and resurfacing with an Integra® regeneration template in a two-stage procedure.

D. Sequential dermabrasion of entire sections of the face (lower, middle, upper third) and application of sheets of medium thickness skin using tissue glue and steri-strip fixation and no sutures.

E. Use the carbon dioxide laser to remove the textural abnormality and immediately apply a cell suspension of keratinocytes harvested from the scalp.

10 When considering extensive burn scarring restricting movement of all joints of both upper limbs, which should be the order of priority for surgical release?

A. The dominant hand should be treated first.

B. The most severely deformed hand should be treated first, irrespective of dominance.

C. The least deformed hand should be treated first, irrespective of dominance.

D. The axilla of the dominant hand should be treated first.

E. The patient should be allowed to choose which joint should be treated first.

11 Indications for removal of teeth in the line of a mandibular fracture include:

A. Gross mobility of the tooth.
B. Root fracture.
C. Exposed apices.
D. None of the above.
E. All of the above.

12 Which two of the following statements are true regarding pigmentary changes following burn injury?

A. Following burn injury hypopigmentation is seen more often than hyperpigmentation.
B. Post-burn hypopigmentation will usually resolve in time.
C. Post-burn hyperpigmentation is a form of post-inflammatory hyperpigmentation and usually responds to a combination of 4% hydroquinine, 0.05% retinoic acid and 0.25% triamcilone acetonide in a cream base.
D. Small areas of post-burn vitiligo can be treated with dermabrasion and application of melanocyte cultures.
E. The only certain way of removing hyperpigmented skin grafts is to excise them and re-graft and insist on complete abstinence from sun exposure.

13 Cyanide poisoning:

A. Is common after chemical burns.
B. Is fatal at concentrations of 1 part per million.
C. Can be treated with amyl nitrite, sodium nitrite and sodium thiosulphate or hydroxycobalamin.
D. Can be treated with ethyl chloride and alkalinisation of urine.
E. Can be treated by 100% oxygen, ethyl chloride and thiopentone.

14 Which one of the following statements do you think would have the greatest consensus support from a panel of international burns experts?

A. Following a deep head and neck burn with loss of the ear and an extensive peri-auricular scar it is possible to use tissue expansion in combination with a superficial temporoparietal fascial turnover flap to create a reasonable ear reconstruction.

B. When both upper and lower eyelids are involved in a scar, the lower lid should be replaced with a full thickness graft as it has less mobility and acts like a dam, while the upper lid is very mobile and a thin, split thickness graft should be used.

C. Following deep perineal burns in the very young male child it may be more appropriate to consider gender reassignment than attempt genital reconstruction which is fraught with difficulties.

D. The greatest challenge of the complex post-burn reconstruction is to match the reconstructive need with the potential donor tissue as every patient has a different pattern of scarring and deformity.

E. Where resources are limited the priority for reconstruction should aim for independent mobility in children, while in adults optimising manual dexterity should be the most important goal.

15 With regards to arm fasciotomies, which one is true?

A. The anterior compartment is decompressed using a lateral incision.

B. The lateral compartment is decompressed using a lateral incision.

C. The posterior compartment is decompressed using a lateral incision.

D. The ulnar nerve can be decompressed simply through a medial incision.

E. The radial nerve can be decompressed simply through a lateral incision.

16 With regard to post-burn reconstruction of the female breast, which of the following statements is correct?

A. Breast development can still occur despite loss of the breast bud prior to puberty.
B. When Integra® is used in the peripubertal stage for release of contractures of the breast skin envelope, the breast can subsequently develop as normal in terms of both volume and ptosis.
C. Because of the tendency for Integra® to contract it is not advisable to use it to release breast contractures as it prevents normal breast development.
D. Tissue expansion should not be used in post-burn breast reconstruction because of the risk of ischaemic damage to the delicate breast bud.
E. It is not possible to breast feed after breast reconstruction in a burns patient.

17 In the primary treatment of burns:

A. Non-sterile cling-film must not be used as a primary dressing.
B. Luke-warm water should be used for first aid.
C. Primary dressings should be removed to allow accurate weighing of patients for calculation of fluid for resuscitation.
D. Antibiotics should be given prophylactically on admission but after swabs have been taken.
E. Consent should be taken from relatives or next of kin before escharotomies are undertaken.

18 In the primary treatment of burns:

A. The first priority is to assess the percentage surface area of burn.
B. The first priority is to provide initial basic fluid resuscitation.
C. Once fluid resuscitation has commenced, other trauma should be excluded.

D.   A 30% partial thickness burn injury with combined severe head injury (Glasgow Coma Scale 7) should initially be managed by neurosurgeons if combined care is not available.
E.   Singed nasal hair should prompt immediate intubation.

19 With regards to burns:

A.   In a child of 10 years, each leg approximates 14% body surface area.
B.   Tangential excision was first described in 1957.
C.   Lightning strikes cause classical cutaneous Lichtenstein figures.

D.   Carbon monoxide has a half-life of approximately 4 hours breathing room air but just over 1 hour breathing 100% oxygen.
E.   The specific antidote for cyanide poisoning is activated charcoal.

20 The following are true about the Le Fort 2 fracture pattern:

A.   It passes across the nasal bones.
B.   It passes through the pterygoid plates.
C.   The bony fragment contains the lacrimal crests and alveolus.
D.   None of the choices.
E.   All of the choices.

21 The following is true regarding Y to V-plasty reconstruction for scar contractures:

A.   Because the tips of the flaps are only undermined a small amount, there is less risk of necrosis of these tips.
B.   The flaps can be re-advanced if contracture recurs.
C.   Flap tip necrosis is more common than with Z-plasty, but the design is simpler.
D.   It is not an ideal technique for contractures longer than approximately 10cm.
E.   None of these is true.

22 The following is the best surgical option to restore dorsiflexion in isolated loss of tibialis anterior function with footdrop with normal soft tissues:

A. This is not a treatable condition.
B. A foot drop splint.
C. Tibialis posterior to tibialis anterior transfer.
D. Ankle fusion in the position of function.
E. Free functioning muscle transfer.

23 With regards to forearm fasciotomies, which one is true?

A. A single, straight-line incision all the way along the ulnar and volar aspect of the forearm is a well-recognised approach for the volar fasciotomy.
B. Mannitol must be used adjunctively because the risk of disabling contracture is so high.
C. It is not possible to decompress both the carpal tunnel and Guyon's canal through the same palmar incision.
D. Hyperbaric oxygen should never be used.
E. None of the above is true.

24 Which of the following is not a criterion for transfer of a burns patient to a specialist burns centre?

A. 25% total body surface area (TBSA) deep partial thickness burns.
B. High voltage electrical burn.
C. 15% TBSA superficial partial thickness burn in a 3-year-old.
D. 20% TBSA superficial only burns.
E. Full thickness burns to the whole of one hand.

25 Which of the following is not a function of skin?

A. Thermoregulatory.
B. Immunological.
C. Vitamin E synthesis.
D. Physical barrier.
E. Ultraviolet protection.

26 The critical zones of injury in a burn that can be influenced by early effective management include:

A. Zone of coagulative necrosis.
B. Zone of hyperaemia.
C. Zone of stasis.
D. A and C.
E. B and C.

27 With respect to paediatric burns which of the following is true?

A. They have lower energy needs.
B. They have thicker skin.
C. They have a larger surface area to body mass ratio.
D. Renal concentrating ability is better than an adult.
E. Hypertrophic scarring is less common.

28 With regards to burn excision:

A. Fascial excision provides excellent cosmesis.
B. The technique of tangential excision was published by Janzekovic in 1970.
C. Fascial excision leads to significant blood loss.
D. Late excision after antimicrobial dressings have been applied for a number of weeks leads to better outcomes.
E. None of the above.

29 Issues relating to local flaps in the reconstruction of traumatic lower limb injuries:

A. The lateral head of gastrocnemius is larger than the medial head.
B. Use of the medial head of gastrocnemius leads to a significant functional deficit
C. Use of a proximally based soleus flap leads to a significant functional deficit.
D. Scoring of the fascia of gastrocnemius can allow the flap to cover a larger area.
E. Soleus and gastrocnemius have the same pattern of vascular supply.

30 The ideal skin substitute would be:

A. Resistant to shear stresses.
B. Toxic.
C. Inelastic.
D. Antigenic.
E. Epidermal only.

31 The following are formulae specifically for calculating nutritional requirements and supplementation after burn injury except for:

A. Curreri formula.
B. Harris-Benedict formula.
C. Galveston Junior formula.
D. Ireton-Jones formula.
E. Davies formula.

32 The following fluid rescucitation is suitable for a 12kg child with 8% burns:

A. 46ml of human albumin solution.
B. 384ml per 24 hours for Parkland's formula of crystalloid.

C.   48ml of normal saline for the first period using Muir and Barclay's regime.
D.   200ml over 24 hours of hypertonic saline.
E.   300ml over 24 hours of human albumin solution (HAS) maintenance.

33 Which one answer is true regarding osteomyelitis in the lower limb?

A.   The commonest causative organism overall is *Streptococcus pyogenes.*

B.   A common causative organism in relation to joint replacements is a common skin commensal.
C.   Is classified by Pairolero.
D.   The incidence in severe open tibial fractures is reduced from almost 50% to <1% with prophylactic antibiotics.
E.   None of the above.

34 The best modality for diagnosis of osteomyelitis is:

A.   MRI.
B.   Combined MRI with CT.
C.   CT.
D.   Bone scan.
E.   Bone biopsy.

35 In the context of acute trauma, permissive hypotension:

A.   Has been universally embraced in the context of acute trauma management by ATLS®.
B.   Describes the process whereby the airway is protected and the C-spine immobilised while the circulation may nevertheless be compromised in the priority sequence 'A, B, C....'.
C.   Is created by the infusion of dopamine.

D.	Involves withholding fluid resuscitation in acute trauma in order to avoid overall blood loss and coagulopathy, which may improve prognosis in patients not *in extremis*.
E.	None of the above is true.

36 The following mechanism is not a recognised cause of compartment syndrome:

A.	Intensive muscle use including vigorous exercise.
B.	Envenomation (e.g. snake, spider).
C.	Nephrotic syndrome.
D.	Everyday exercise activities such as cycling, horseriding.
E.	Giant lipoma.

37 The following is the best indication for lower limb fasciotomy:

A.	Full thickness electrical burn to the left leg of 12% body surface area.
B.	Compartment pressures of 15mmHg.
C.	Compartment pressures of 20mmHg.
D.	Positive Homan's sign.
E.	Negative Homan's sign.

Section 5 answers

Burns and trauma

1 D.

Reconstructive burn surgery should begin in the acute burn phase. If there is a functional problem, early intervention is appropriate. Children do pose special problems because of the additional dimension of growth. In these circumstances flaps are usually better than grafts and there is certainly no need to wait until growth stops. Burn reconstruction is aimed at both function and form, and deals with far more than contractures and mobility. We must always be thinking of the reconstructive outcome when we are dealing with acute burns. Appropriately treated, no further reconstruction may be needed despite extensive, deep burns.

2 D.

Increased pulmonary vascular resistance.

3 D.

Eyes, mouth, scalp, nose, ears. Prioritizing is very important in reconstructive burns surgery and the concept of a 'shopping list' of problems is well established. In terms of anatomy, it is possible to look at problems objectively or, in terms of the patient's perception of disability and deformity, it is possible to look at problems subjectively. In this question, we are focusing on the head and neck with involvement of a number of anatomical features. When we consider prioritizing the reconstructive strategy we have to look at the seriousness of the consequence(s) of the scarring and in this context the loss of vision must be considered the number one complication to avoid. The second complication of greatest significance would be loss of oral continence if there is lip ectropion or poor feeding and vocalisation if there is microstomia. There will always be debate about the priority of the other features but a general consensus would agree with eyes first, mouth second.

4 E.

Integra® is a bilaminar biodegradable tissue engineered dermal matrix generation template. Integra® does not inherently contract. It is physically inert, but placed in a flexor recipient site without postoperative rehabilitation and the newly generated auto-collagenous dermal matrix will contract. Of note, Integra® contains chondroitin-6-sulphate, does not cause infection but can become infected, and does not act as a template for skin regeneration.

References
1.   Young RC, Burd A. Paediatric upper limb contracture release following burn injury. *Burns* 2004; 30(7): 723-8.

5 D.

Where the technical skills and resources exist there are relatively few patients who can benefit from the surgery. Sadly, in much of the developing world where the need for resources and expertise is much greater, many such children struggle to survive.

References
1.   Burd A, Pang PCW, Ying SY, Ayyappan T. Microsurgical reconstruction in children's burns. *J Plast Reconstr Aesthet Surg* 2006; 59: 679-92.

6 E.

None of the above. The medial and dorsal approaches are commonly used. The medial approach affords access to all four compartments of the foot and is made along the plantar border of the first metatarsal. The dorsal approach involves two incisions along the second and fourth interspaces.

References

1. Broughton, G II. Compartment syndrome. In: *Essentials of plastic surgery handbook: a UT Southwestern Medical Center handbook.* Janis JE. St. Louis, USA: Quality Medical Publishing Inc., 2007: 634.

7 C.

25kcal/kg + 40kcal/% burn. The calculation is undertaken as follows: 25kcal x usual body weight in kilograms + 40 x % total body surface area burned. This is the Curreri formula (adult). For children, the formula is 60kcal/kg + 35kcal/% burn. Feeding should be given enterally when possible and the decision between naso-enteral feeding or a formal jejunostomy will depend on patient factors and ideally commence within 24 hours of admission for major burns. Many other formulae also exist, and there is no consensus as to the best regime.

8 D.

The motivation and compliance of the patient (and/or parents). One can be an excellent surgeon but achieve poor outcomes if there is no program of postoperative rehabilitation. Equally, excellent surgeons with good postoperative rehabilitation teams can still have poor outcomes if patients are poorly motivated. In nearly every case of excellent functional outcome in the field of post-burn reconstruction you will find a highly motivated patient. The converse is also true and so patient selection is very important.

9 D.

Sequential dermabrasion of entire sections of the face (lower, middle, upper third) and application of sheets of medium thickness skin using tissue glue and steri-strip fixation and no sutures. As in many aspects of reconstructive surgery there will be individuals who have a strong preference for certain strategies. In this question the problem of extensive textural abnormality is the focus of concern. As such, any extensive full thickness skin/scar excision will carry a significant risk of scarring secondary to infection and impaired healing. The alternative is to keep the bulk of the dermal matrix and to flatten the textural abnormality with dermabrasion or ablative laser therapy. Mechanical dermabrasion does carry health risks because of the associated aerosol spray but the use of protective masks and screens can prevent contamination. Using sequential dermabrasion of entire sections of the face and applying intact sheets of medium thickness graft and using an atraumatic fixation technique, optimal results can be achieved.

10 D.

The axilla of the dominant hand should be treated first. The hand is unable to function without restoration first of proximal mobility, and the dominant limb is a priority. There is no point in performing complicated reconstructive surgery in the hand of an immobile upper limb. The principle is to work from trunk to extremity and in the upper limb consider the sequential release of axilla, elbow, wrist then hand and prioritizing the side that will give the dominant hand optimum function.

References
1.   Young RC, Burd A. Paediatric upper limb contracture release following burn injury. *Burns* 2004; 30(7): 723-8.

11 E.

All of the above. All of these are indications for extraction.

References
1.   Potter JK. Facial skeletal trauma (adult/pediatric). In: *Essentials of plastic surgery.* Janis JE. St Louis, USA: Quality Medical Publishing Inc., 2007: 251.

12 D and E.

Small areas of post-burn vitiligo can be treated with dermabrasion and application of melanocyte cultures and *the only certain way of removing hyperpigmented skin grafts is to excise them and re-graft and insist on complete abstinence from sun exposure.* Pigmentary changes following burns can be particularly distressing in dark skinned patients. Post-burn vitiligo can have adverse cultural stigmata. Overall, hyperpigmentation is more often seen particularly in grafts. It is not a post-inflammatory problem in many cases and can be difficult to resolve. There are reports of successful treatment of small areas of stable vitiligo with dermabrasion and application of melanocyte (containing) cell culture.

References
1.   Grover R, Morgan BD. Management of hypopigmentation following burn injury. *Burns* 1996; 22(8): 627-30.

159

13 c.

Can be treated with amyl nitrite, sodium nitrite and sodium thiosulphate or hydroxycobalamin. Cyanide poisoning can rapidly cause death. Having an effective antidote readily available is essential for facilities that provide emergency care. In cases of cyanide ingestion, both the nitrite/thiosulphate combination and hydroxycobalamin are effective antidotes. Hydroxycobalamin offers an improved safety profile for children and pregnant women. Hydroxycobalamin also appears to have a better safety profile in the setting of cyanide poisoning in conjunction with smoke inhalation. However, current data are insufficient to recommend the empiric administration of hydroxycobalamin to all victims of smoke inhalation.

References
1.   Shepherd G, Velez LI. Role of hydroxycobalamin in acute cyanide poisoning. *Ann Pharmacother* 2008; 42(5): 661-9.

14 d.

The greatest challenge of the complex post-burn reconstruction is to match the reconstructive need with the potential donor tissue as every patient has a different pattern of scarring and deformity. The management of burns has a good grounding in 'experience-based medicine'. Ear reconstruction is a considerable challenge with healthy peri-auricular tissue. In the presence of scarring it becomes very difficult and many experts would simply not embark on autologous reconstruction particularly if osteointegration and prosthetic support is available. Thin split thickness grafts should not be used as upper eyelids. The grafts will contract and problems will recur. Genital reconstruction is extremely challenging particularly when donor sites are limited but there are experts who can perform such surgery. Appropriate referral for such reconstruction would be much more preferable than the alternative of 'forcing' gender reassignment. The goals of reconstruction in children and adults can differ but generally functional independence is the theme. The statement, however, which is least controversial relates to the challenge of the match of donor tissue to recipient sites. The individual and specific nature of the scarring of burn patients may require radically different reconstructive strategies in two patients who have similar functional problems to address.

15 C.

The posterior compartment is decompressed using a lateral incision. The anterior compartment is decompressed using a medial incision. There is no lateral compartment in the arm. The radial and ulnar nerves travel in both compartments for part of their course, so medial and lateral incisions to decompress both compartments are needed to decompress each one of these nerves.

References

1.   Velmahos GC, Toutouzas KG. Vascular trauma and compartment syndromes. *Surg Clin N Am* 2002; 82: 125

16 B.

When Integra® is used in the peripubertal stage for release of contractures of the breast skin envelope, the breast can subsequently develop as normal in terms of both volume and ptosis. In the *International Hand Book* published by Integra Life Sciences, a case of breast contracture release in an adolescent girl with 6 years follow-up demonstrates that by using Integra® a new cover could be achieved for the breast that could accommodate normal breast development both in size and shape. An important element of this reconstruction was the preservation of the breast bud because without this a breast could not develop. Breast feeding is still possible after post-burn breast reconstruction. It will depend on an intact ductal system and functioning nipple. A very effective way of releasing contractures distorting the breasts and resurfacing areas of the breast is to use tissue expansion.

17 B.

Luke-warm water should be used for first aid. The specific heat capacity of water is high and it is thus very efficient at removing heat energy. Overly cold first aid is detrimental as it causes reflex vasoconstriction leading to further tissue ischaemia and potentially increasing the extent of the injury in areas of borderline viability.

18 D.

A 30% partial thickness burn injury with combined severe head injury (Glasgow Coma Scale 7) should initially be managed by neurosurgeons if combined care is not available. The first priority is to assess and maintain the airway and breathing with due attention to the cervical spine.

19 A.

In a child of 10 years, each leg approximates 14% body surface area. Tangential excision was developed by Zora Janzekovic in the late 1960s and published in 1970. Lightning strike causes characteristic Lichtenberg figures. The half-life on room air is 4 hours but is 45 minutes breathing 100% oxygen, and this is reduced to 30 minutes with hyperbaric oxygen. Specfic antidotes for cyanide poisoning include a combination of amyl nitrite, sodium nitrite and sodium thiosulphate, or hydroxycobalamin.

References

1.   Janzekovic Z. A new concept in the early excision and immediate grafting of burns. *J Trauma* 1970; 10(12): 1103-8.

20 E.

All of the choices. All of these are true. These fracture patterns are well described and widely reproduced (Figure 1).

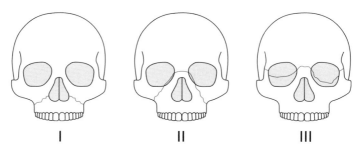

Figure 1. Le Fort 2 fracture patterns.

21 B.

The flaps can be re-advanced if contracture recurs. The Y to V-plasty technique is a versatile technique. There is no undermining at all of the flap tips which makes the flaps robust - more so than Z-plasty flaps, and they can be re-advanced. Long lengths of contracture can be released.

22 C.

Tibialis posterior to tibialis anterior transfer. TP to TA transfer is a useful technique. Splintage is not a surgical technique nor does it restore dorsiflexion. Ankle fusion does not restore dorsiflexion. Free functioning muscle transfer is too complex a procedure in comparison to TPTA transfer, has significant donor morbidity, and will not provide as successful a reconstruction where soft tissues are uninjured.

23 A.

A single, straight-line incision all the way along the ulnar and volar aspect of the forearm is a well-recognised approach for the volar fasciotomy. A single ulnar volar incision is a reasonable choice for volar fasciotomy. The Lazy-S incision is anecdotally more popular nevertheless. Mannitol has shown promise as an adjunct, but has not entered routine practice. Hyperbaric oxygen has shown considerable promise as an adjunct, but is limited in its use by availability, cost and transfer issues.

References

1.   Broughton G II. Compartment syndrome. In: *Essentials of plastic surgery handbook: a UT Southwestern Medical Center handbook*. Janis JE. St. Louis, USA: Quality Medical Publishing Inc., 2007: 634.

24 D.

20% TBSA superficial only burns. D is not a criterion. Referral should be made of all major partial or full thickness burns in adults (>10%TBSA), any childhood burns of concern, and burns to unique areas (hand, genitalia, face), although these criteria vary slightly by country and jurisdiction. High voltage electrical burns with the potential for major internal burn injuries are also included. Superficial only burns are not included when calculating TBSA.

25 C.

Vitamin E synthesis. The skin synthesises Vitamin D, not E. Vitamin E is a component of many moisturisers however.

26 E.

B and C. B and C are correct. The zone of coagulative necrosis is non-viable, and thus not reversible, while the zones of hyperaemia and stasis are potentially salvageable. Early burns management is aimed at preventing the progression of the potentially viable zones into coagulative necrosis. These zones were described by Jackson.

References

1.   Jackson DM. The diagnosis of the depth of burning. *Br J Surg* 1952; 40: 566-96.

27 C.

They have a larger surface area to body mass ratio. Children have higher energy needs, thinner skin, and immature kidneys. While healing is quicker in children, the incidence of hypertrophic scarring is greater. Children also have a larger surface area to body mass ratio.

28 B.

The technique of tangential excision was published by Janzekovic in 1970. Zora Janzekovic published her technique of tangential excision for burns in 1970. Fascial excision leads to reduced blood loss compared with tangential excision, but at the cost of poor cosmesis depending on the area involved. Early burn excision leads to improved outcomes.

References

1. Janzekovic Z. A new concept in the early excision and immediate grafting of burns. *J Trauma* 1970; 10(12): 1103-8.

29 D.

Scoring of the fascia of gastrocnemius can allow the flap to cover a larger area. Scoring of the gastrocnemius fascia extends the potential area of cover and reach. The medial head of gastrocnemius is bigger than the lateral. Each of gastrocnemius and soleus muscles is expendable without undue donor functional morbidity. The pattern of vascular supply for each head of gastrocnemius is Type I, and for soleus Type II.

References

1. Mathes SJ, Nahai F. *Reconstructive surgery: principles, anatomy & technique.* New York, USA: Churchill Livingstone, 1997.

30 A.

Resistant to shear stresses. A skin substitute would require adherence to the wound bed (resistant to shear stresses), not be rejected (non-toxic, non-antigenic) and function as skin (elastic and have all components of skin including dermis).

31 B.

Harris-Benedict formula. All except the Harris-Benedict formula specifically calculate nutritional requirements after burns. The Harris-Benedict formula calculates basal calorific requirements. However, it can still be used in the calculation of nutritional requirements by multiplying the basal requirements by a stress factor which usually ranges between 1.2 and 1.8 depending on severity of burn. The Curreri formula was developed retrospectively based upon just nine cases.

32 B.

384ml per 24 hours for Parkland's formula of crystalloid.

33 B.

A common causative organism in relation to joint replacements is a common skin commensal. A common causative organism in relation to joint replacements is *Staphylococcus epidermidis*. The commonest organism overall is *S. aureus*. Pairolero discussed osteomyelitis of the sternum. The incidence of infection in severe tibial fractures using antibiotic prophylaxis is reduced from 24% to 4%.

References
1.   Patzakis MJ Wilkins J. Moore TM. Use of antibiotics in open tibial fractures. *Clin Orthop Relat Res* 1983; 178: 31-5.

34 E.

Bone biopsy. Imaging modalities may show subtle changes early in the course of osteomyelitis, but often does not. Bone biopsy provides not only a definitive diagnosis of infection, but differentiates from other causes including tumours.

35 D.

Involves withholding fluid resuscitation in acute trauma in order to avoid overall blood loss and coagulopathy, which may improve prognosis in patients not in extremis. Although not universally accepted, some trauma centres are moving towards acceptance of the concept of permissive hypotension. This concept allows moderate hypotension in the context of acute trauma because early aggressive fluid resuscitation can increase overall blood loss and causes clotting abnormalities. It is yet to be embraced by ATLS® at the time of writing (2009).

36 E.

Giant lipoma. This is not a recognised cause of compartment syndrome. Compartment syndrome can be caused by increased interstitial volume or decreased compartmental space. All the options listed except lipoma are recognised causes due to an increased interstitial pressure - as are haemorrhage, and severe burns. Everyday exercise activities can very rarely also cause compartment syndrome which is well documented in the literature. A decrease in compartment size can also be due to burns, as well as the use of cast splints, prolonged lying on a limb and use of military anti-shock trousers (MAST).

References

1.   Broughton, G II. Compartment syndrome. In: *Essentials of plastic surgery handbook: a UT Southwestern Medical Center handbook.* Janis JE. St. Louis, USA: Quality Medical Publishing Inc., 2007: 634.

37 A.

Full thickness electrical burn to the left leg of 12% body surface area. Homan's sign was described in the context of deep venous thrombosis and has been largely discredited due to poor specificity and sensitivity as a clinical sign. Compartment pressure monitoring is controversial and the leg has four compartments that can have variable pressures in each. A high index of suspicion in the context of history and clinical examination in the scenario of an electrical injury of this nature would warrant fasciotomy.

Section 6 questions

Reconstructive head and neck surgery

1 Which is true concerning reconstruction of the eyelids?

A. The Mustardé flap and the Tenzel flap are equivalent.
B. Defects of up to 50% may be closed primarily with the addition of a canthotomy and cantholysis.
C. Defects greater than 75% are unreconstructable.
D. The Tripier flap is a single stage bilobed flap suitable for reconstruction of the entire lower eyelid.
E. Defects of up to 75% may be closed primarily with the addition of a canthotomy and cantholysis.

2 Frey's syndrome:

A. Occurs in approximately 50% of patients following a submandibular gland excision.
B. Occurs when parasympathetic innervation of sweat glands is replaced by sympathetic innervation to the parotid gland.
C. Botulinum toxin is licensed for use in its symptomatic treatment.
D. Was described by Lucja Frey-Gottesman in the 8th century.
E. Is also known as Baillarger's syndrome.

3   Sensory nerves to the ear include all except:

A.   Auricular branch of vagus.
B.   Superficial temporal nerve.
C.   Auriculotemporal nerve.
D.   Lesser occipital nerve.
E.   Great auricular nerve.

4   With regards to the eyes and eyelids, which statement is correct?

A.   The lacrimal gland secretes tears which are bilaminar, consisting of a superficial mucoprotein layer and a deep aqueous layer.
B.   The lacrimal gland has three lobes.
C.   Tears bend incoming light before it strikes the cornea with up to 2.0 diopters of refractile power.
D.   The superior tarsal plate is 8-10mm in vertical height and the inferior tarsal plate is smaller at 4-6mm.
E.   The lacrimal sac is situated above and medial to the lateral canthus.

5   In relation to pharyngoplasty:

A.   Hynes' procedure is a posterior wall technique.
B.   Orticochea described a posterior wall technique.
C.   Lateral wall techniques can result in snoring and respiratory obstruction.
D.   Inferiorly-based techniques involve elevation of a flap that is inset into the hard palate.
E.   Nasendoscopy with contrast medium can help assess suitability for surgery.

6   Which one of the following is considered a non-immunologic-related complication of immuno-suppression in face transplantation?

A.   Acute rejection.
B.   Opportunistic infection.
C.   Malignancy.
D.   Nephrotoxicity.
E.   All of the above are considered immunologic-related complications.

7   Split ear lobes are caused by all except (choose 2):

A.   Heavy earrings.
B.   Anorexia.
C.   Obesity.
D.   Metal allergy.
E.   Trauma.

8   Which one of the following immunosuppressives is believed to promote nerve regeneration in face transplantation?

A.   Mycophenolate mofetil.
B.   Tacrolimus.
C.   Cyclosporine.
D.   Rapamycin.
E.   Steroids.

9   The progression rate of oral leukoplakia to invasive cancer within at least 12 years is:

A.   30%.
B.   40%.
C.   50%.
D.   60-100%.
E.   None of the above.

10 Which of the following is the most common malignancy due to immunosuppression in transplant recipients?

A.   Lymphoproliferative.
B.   Skin cancer.
C.   Kaposi's sarcoma.
D.   Renal cell carcinoma.
E.   Brain tumor.

11 A 37-year-old woman is undergoing evaluation because of intermittent locking of the right temporomandibular joint (TMJ). She has no pain or crepitus of the joint. Interincisal opening is 40mm. MRI shows a non-reducing articular disk within the right TMJ. Which of the following is the most appropriate management?

A.   Observation.
B.   Intracapsular repositioning of the disk.
C.   Intracapsular repositioning of the disk and reduction of the articular eminence.
D.   Removal of the disk and placement of an interpositional temporalis fascia flap.
E.   Manipulation under anaesthesia (MUA) followed by splintage.

12 Maxillary sinus tumours:

A. Some tumours may be accessed using a Webster-Fergusohn incision.
B. Orbital exenteration is almost never required.
C. The wider and higher the defect the greater the likelihood that a free flap will be required for reconstruction.
D. A DCIA flap will not provide sufficient bony stock for restorative dentistry implant rehabilitation.
E. Biopsy is not usually indicated prior to tumour surgery in view of the destructive nature of exposure required to sample any suspicious lesion.

13 The following are risk factors associated with the malignant transformation of leukoplakia except:

A. Long duration.
B. Gender (women > men).
C. Idiopathic leukoplakia (i.e. occurring in non-smokers).
D. Presence of *Candida albicans*.
E. Location on the buccal mucosa (as opposed to the floor of the mouth or tongue).

14 A 24-year-old woman undergoes a LeFort I osteotomy with maxillary impaction and bilateral sagittal split osteotomy with mandibular advancement. Following release of intermaxillary fixation 6 weeks later, the patient has an anterior open bite. Which of the following is the most likely cause of this finding?

A. Improper intra-operative seating of the condyles in the glenoid fossae.
B. Improper presurgical orthodontic treatment.
C. Loosening of all plates of the rigid internal fixation.
D. Parafunctional habits, such as tongue thrusting.
E. Progressive resorption of the condyles.

15 A patient has an infection at the surgical site 1 week after undergoing open reduction and internal fixation of a fracture of the mandibular body using an inferior border reconstruction plate and a tension band. Occlusion is normal. The infection site is surgically drained; intra-operative exploration shows that the plates and screws are stable with no evidence of loosening. Which of the following is the most appropriate management of the hardware?

A.   Removal of all plates and immediate application of intermaxillary fixation.
B.   Removal of all plates and immediate application of two miniplates.
C.   Removal of all plates and immediate placement of an external fixator.
D.   Removal of all plates and placement of new plates when the infection has subsided.
E.   None of these.

16 A 32-year-old woman has near complete paralysis of the lower portion of the left side of the face 3 years after onset of Bell's palsy. There has been no return of nerve function for the past year. Examination shows adequate function of the orbicularis oculi muscle and a good Bell's reflex. Which of the following is the most appropriate management?

A.   Continued observation.
B.   Hypoglossal nerve transfer.
C.   Placement of a gold weight in the eyelid and static brow lifting.
D.   Neurotized free muscle transfer using innervation from cross-face grafts.
E.   Temporalis muscle transfer to the upper and lower eyelids.

17 Calcification of the ear occurs in all except (choose 2):

A. Frostbite injuries.
B. Neurofibromata.
C. Keloids.
D. Acrobatic ears.
E. Otohaematoma.

18 A 7-year-old has cryptotia. Which of the following operative techniques is most appropriate for correction?

A. Advancement of the third crus of the antihelix.
B. Partial detachment of the folded segment of helical cartilage from the scapha and repositioning of the helix with sutures.
C. Placement of sutures from the conchal bowl to the mastoid fascia.
D. Rasping of the anterior surface of the antihelical cartilage to create the antihelix.
E. Separation of the superior auricle from the temporal skin with placement of a retro-auricular skin graft.

19 With regards to tracheostomies:

A. A Bjork flap is an inferiorly-based U-shaped flap of anterior tracheal wall.
B. It is best to enter the trachea above the first cartilaginous ring.
C. The tracheal rings are located between the thyroid cartilage and the manubrium.
D. The parathyroid glands need to be seen and preserved during the procedure.
E. They are bloodless midline operative procedures.

20 Concerning acute rejection in composite tissue transplantation, which one of the following statements is incorrect?

A. Is primarily T-cell-mediated.
B. Is reversible in almost all cases.
C. Topical immunosuppressives have no role in its treatment.
D. Is characterised by perivascular infiltration of lymphocytes in the upper and mid dermis.
E. There is a high correlation between clinical and histopathological findings of acute rejection.

21 A 30-year-old woman is undergoing examination 6 months after sustaining peri-orbital lacerations in a motor vehicle collision. She has 3.5mm of ptosis, and her levator function is greater than 10mm. Which of the following is the most appropriate management?

A. Advancement of Müller's muscle.
B. Eyebrow suspension.
C. Fasanella-Servat procedure.
D. Repositioning/repair of the levator aponeurosis.
E. Levator resection.

22 The projection of a normal ear (rim-mastoid distance) is:

A. 9mm.
B. 19mm.
C. 29mm.
D. 39mm.
E. None of the above.

6 Reconstructive head and neck surgery

23 Based on current knowledge which of the following is a better estimate of the risk of acute rejection of the facial flap in facial transplantation?

A.   5-10%.
B.   20-50%.
C.   10-70%.
D.   80-90%.
E.   100%.

24 Regarding MRI in the investigation of head and neck cancer:

A.   Is capable of identifying all enlarged nodes greater than 4-5mm in diameter.
B.   Can differentiate between benign and malignant lymphadenopathy.
C.   Is inferior diagnostically to traditional clinical examination.
D.   Is superior to CT for assessing bony involvement.
E.   T2-weighted images may slightly underestimate lymph node size.

25 Regarding reconstruction/excision of tumours of the oral cavity:

A.   Pedicled flaps are more reliable than free flaps.
B.   Soutar described the use of the radial forearm flap in oral cavity reconstruction.
C.   The soft palate is in the oral cavity.
D.   Always requires a free flap.
E.   Mandibular splits should be performed lateral to the first molar tooth.

26 Which two of the following anatomic structures of the ear originates from the second (hyoid) pharyngeal arch?

A. Antitragus.
B. Helical root.
C. Superior helix.
D. Tragus.
E. Lobule.

27 The following portion of a histopathological report most likely refers to which pathology?: "A sparse chronic inflammatory infiltrate is seen with small blood vessels arranged perpendicular to the skin surface. Glassy collagen is seen. Immunohistochemistry reveals smooth muscle actin in a tram-track pattern with scattered S-100 positive cells. Desmin is negative."

A. Melanoma.
B. Squamous carcinoma.
C. Basal carcinoma.
D. Hypertrophic/keloid scar.
E. None of the above.

28 Concerning tumours of the paranasal sinuses:

A. Nasal polyps have a 2% malignant potential.
B. Are mainly adenocarcinoma.
C. Most commonly present in the <50-year age group.
D. Are commonest in Western Europe.
E. Commonly metastasize to lymph nodes.

29 The paramedian forehead flap receives its blood supply from:

A.   The supratrochlear vessels.
B.   The supra-orbital vessels.
C.   Vessels continuing from the angular branch of the facial artery.
D.   A and C.
E.   B and C.

30 Raising of the paramedian forehead flap:

A.   Should allow for primary closure of the donor site.
B.   Needs a tissue expander in larger defects to close the donor site.
C.   Needs a skin graft to close the donor site.
D.   Should leave the donor site open and allow healing by secondary intention.
E.   Is never a problem as the pedicle is generally placed back to the forehead after division.

31 The anterolateral thigh flap shows a septocutaneous blood supply in approximately:

A.   10%.
B.   30%.
C.   50%.
D.   70%.
E.   90%.

32 A floppy ear, lacking in stiffness, is seen in (choose 2):

A.   Newborn infants.
B.   Frostbite.
C.   Rugby players.
D.   Teenagers.
E.   Relapsing polychondritis.

33 The following is not in the left supraclavicular triangle of the neck:

A. Inferior cervical lymph nodes.
B. Subclavian artery.
C. Thoracic duct.
D. Phrenic nerve.
E. Spinal accessory nerve.

34 Concerning head and neck tumours:

A. Squamous cell carcinoma (SCC) is the most common cancer involving the head and neck mucosal sites, accounting for 70% of all malignancies.
B. Drinking and smoking tobacco act synergistically to increase the lifetime risk by a factor of three.
C. Management is best delivered in a multidisciplinary setting.
D. There are five lymphatic drainage levels.
E. Magnetic resonance imaging is too expensive for use for investigation.

35 Before starting microsurgery the microscope should be prepared by:

A. No special necessary tests.
B. Zooming out to least magnification and focusing till the picture is sharp.
C. Zooming in to most magnification and focusing till the picture is sharp.
D. Zooming to the level you want to work at and focusing till the picture is sharp.
E. Switching it off for 10 seconds to cancel any potential magnetism of instruments.

36 The male ear (choose 2):

A.   Is approximately 58mm long.
B.   Is approximately 68mm long.
C.   Is approximately 78mm long.
D.   Is larger than the female ear.
E.   Decreases in size in old age.

37 To prevent microvascular anastomosis occlusion in a standard microsurgical case you should:

A.   Keep the operating theatre temperature high.
B.   Make sure both vessels are of the same calibre.
C.   Make sure there is no intimal damage in either vessel.
D.   Inject a bolus of heparin before putting the clamp on the vessel.
E.   Never release the vein before starting the arterial anastomosis.

38 The two most likely diagnoses of a painful nodule on the rim of the ear are (choose 2):

A.   Neurofibroma.
B.   Keloid.
C.   Chondrodermatitis.
D.   Basal cell carcinoma.
E.   Gouty tophus.

39 The following cystic tumours of the neck are not appropriately matched to their frequency of occurrence and age of occurrence:

A.   Infant - thyroglossal duct cyst - most frequent.
B.   Adolescent - thyroglossal duct cyst - most frequent.
C.   Adult - thyroglossal duct cyst - most frequent.
D.   Adult - cervical thymic cyst - very uncommon.
E.   Adult - metastatic cystic carcinoma - most frequent.

40 In relation to facial musculature and facial palsy, which one is true?

A. The muscles are composed of four layers.
B. Layer 4 is innervated via its deep surface.
C. Layer 1 is innervated via its superficial surface.
D. Paralysis occurs most commonly due to parotid tumours.
E. Paralysis due to Bell's palsy rarely recovers fully.

41 What method did Sushruta recommend for nasal reconstruction?

A. Scalp flap.
B. Forehead flap.
C. Arm flap.
D. Skin graft.
E. Cheek flap.

42 Microtia is more common in (choose two):

A. Boys.
B. Girls.
C. On the right.
D. On the left.
E. Twins.

43 Which one of the following statements is false regarding head and neck anatomy?

A. Omohyoid originates from the upper border of the scapula and raises the hyoid bone.
B. The blood supply of omohyoid is the inferior thyroid artery.
C. A level III neck dissection involves the removal of nodes which includes the middle jugular group.

D.   Trapezius forms the posterior boundary of a level V neck dissection.
E.   Bocca is often credited as the first to describe the functional neck dissection in the 1960s.

44 T3 N3 M0 SCC of the alveolus of the mandibular symphysis may need the following except:

A.   Free fibular osteocutaneous flap.
B.   Bilateral radical neck dissection with preservation of the left internal jugular vein.
C.   Postoperative radiotherapy.
D.   Marginal mandibulectomy.
E.   Tracheostomy.

45 With regards to ptosis:

A.   It can be treated with Botulinum toxin.
B.   It is associated with mydriasis in Horner's syndrome.
C.   Gold weights are usually adequate treatment.
D.   Muller's muscle may be dysfunctional.
E.   Iatrogenic causes are the leading cause of litigation throughout surgical practice across all specialties.

46 A malignant tumour of the parotid gland:

A.   Is likely to be in the deep lobe.
B.   Is likely to be a metastasis.
C.   Will tend to produce gustatory sweating.
D.   Rarely involves the facial nerve.
E.   Should not be needle-biopsied.

47 What is the major artery in central and lower face transplantation (also referred to as partial facial transplantation)?

A.   Maxillary artery.
B.   Facial artery.
C.   Superior and inferior labial arteries.
D.   Lateral nasal artery.
E.   Superficial temporal artery.

48 Regarding head and neck tumours, which one of the following statements is false?

A.   McFee described the classical 'Y' incision used for neck dissection.
B.   Crile first described the radical neck dissection in 1906.
C.   A tumour limited to the larynx, with vocal cord fixation, an ipsilateral neck node <3cm and no evidence of metastases would be stage 3 disease.
D.   A tumour limited to the vocal cord with normal or impaired mobility and no evidence of nodal spread or distant metastases is stage 2 disease.
E.   A tumour <1cm limited to the subglottis, with no evidence of nodal spread but evidence of distant metastases is stage 4 disease.

49 Which of the following statements is false regarding face transplantation?

A.   The composite flap could be based on the superficial temporal artery.
B.   The composite flap could be based on the facial artery.
C.   Tacrolimus has shown promising results in experimental studies linking it to faster neural regrowth.
D.   Partial face transplants have been performed in France, USA and China.
E.   There have been no recorded mortalities so far following face transplantation.

50 The parotid gland:

A. Develops from the 4th branchial arch.
B. Contains mainly mucous cells.
C. Receives sympathetic supply from the glossopharyngeal nerve via the otic ganglion.
D. Lies deep to the SMAS layer.
E. Stenson's duct empties secretions into the oral cavity opposite the second premolar tooth.

51 Regarding tumour invasion of the mandible from an oral cavity squamous carcinoma:

A. The pathophysiology of mandibular invasion from an oral cancer alters after radiotherapy.
B. Usually leads to decreased sensation in the lip.
C. Makes a tumour inoperable.
D. The best way of determining bony invasion is with a bone scan.
E. A SCC can only invade through the occlusal ridge of the mandible in a dentate patient.

52 Which one of the following is not a recognised cause of facial palsy?

A. AIDS.
B. Guillain-Barré syndrome.
C. Pfeiffer's syndrome.
D. Cholesteatoma.
E. Lyme disease.

53 Neck dissections:

A. There is a proven survival benefit in performing elective neck dissections for thick melanomas (>4mm Breslow thickness) of the head and neck.

B.   A modified radical neck dissection is one in which five lymph nodes of the neck are excised along with the sternomastoid muscle, the spinal accessory nerve and the internal jugular vein.
C.   Air embolus is a common complication of neck dissections.
D.   May lead to a hoarse voice postoperatively.
E.   The marginal mandibular nerve lies superficial to the platysma.

54 Total glossectomy:

A.   A laryngectomy should always be performed at the same time to avoid aspiration.

B.   Patients may be able to speak and swallow after an appropriate reconstruction.
C.   A small thin pliable mobile flap should be used to reconstruct the defect.
D.   Is the treatment of choice for most T2 lateral tongue squamous cell carcinomata.
E.   There is no place in modern head and neck cancer management for such a destructive procedure.

55 Regarding free tissue transfer of the fibula bone:

A.   In adults, the vascular pedicle to the fibula flap is usually limited in length to approximately 12cm.
B.   Arteria peronea magna is a relative contraindication to fibula flap harvest.
C.   The double-barrelled fibula flap configuration was first reported by Jupiter *et al* for long bone reconstruction.
D.   According to Mathes and Nahai, the fibula bone, like the pectoralis muscle, has a Type V vascular pattern.
E.   For mandibular reconstruction, bicortical screw fixation of the osteotomised free fibula is recommended over unicortical fixation for improved stability of the neomandible.

Section 6 answers

Reconstructive head and neck surgery

1   B.

Defects of up to 50% may be closed primarily with the addition of a canthotomy and cantholysis. The Tripier flap is a bipedicled flap suitable for reconstruction of the anterior lamella. Subtotal eyelid defects can be reconstructed in parts, such as with chondromucosal grafts for the posterior lamella and cheek flaps for the anterior lamella. Tenzel and Mustardé described different flaps, the former being a smaller flap based around the outer canthus and the latter a cheek rotation flap.

2   E.

Is also known as Baillarger's syndrome. Frey's syndrome only occurs after surgical procedures on the parotid gland. It occurs when parasympathetic fibres normally destined for the parotid reinnervate the sympathetic receptors of the sweat glands. It can be treated by botulinum toxin but currently there is no licence for this. Although Lucja Frey-Gottesman described the syndrome, it was not in the 8th century and it is also known as Baillarger's syndrome.

3   B.

Superficial temporal nerve.

4   D.

The superior tarsal plate is 8-10 mm in vertical height and the inferior tarsal plate is smaller at 4-6mm. The lacrimal gland secretes a trilaminar layer of tears consisting of a deep mucoprotein layer, a middle aqueous layer and a superficial lipid layer. The lacrimal gland has two lobes, the larger orbital lobe and a smaller palpebral lobe. Tears have a refractive power of up to 0.5 diopters. The lacrimal gland is situated above and medial to the lateral canthus, whereas the lacrimal sac is medial to the medial canthus, posterior to the insertion of the canthal tendon within the lacrimal fossa.

5   C.

Lateral wall techniques can result in snoring and respiratory obstruction.

6   D.

Nephrotoxicity. Immunosuppression-associated risks are divided into two groups: immunologic and non-immunologic. Immunologic-related risks include under-immunosuppression (acute rejection) and over-immunosuppression (opportunistic infections and malignancies). Non-immunologic risks are primarily drug-induced toxicities (e.g. cardiovascular, renal, diabetes). Chronic rejection is considered to be due to a combination of the above two factors.

7   B and C.

Anorexia and *obesity*.

8   B.

Tacrolimus. Tacrolimus is believed to promote nerve regeneration, and therefore has an advantage in composite tissue transplantation of the hands and face, over solid organ transplantation.

9 E.

None of the above. The progression rate to cancer is variably quoted ranging from 2.7% to 17.5%.

References

1.   Gnepp DR. *Diagnostic surgical pathology of the head and neck*, 2nd ed. Saunders-Elsevier, 2009: 9.

10 B.

Skin cancer. Skin cancer is by far the commonest malignancy in organ transplant recipients. The incidence of squamous cell carcinoma (SCC) is reported to be 65 to 250 times higher and that of basal cell carcinoma (BCC) ten times higher in renal transplant recipients when compared with the general population. Other frequently seen cancers are lymphoproliferative disorders, cancers of the pharynx, larynx and oral cavity, and Kaposi sarcoma.

11 A.

Observation.

References

1.   Bays RA. Surgery for internal derangement. In: *Oral and maxillofacial surgery*, 4th ed. Bays RA, Quinn PD, Eds. Philadelphia, USA: Saunders, 2000: 275-300.

2.   Feinberg S, Larsen P. Reconstruction of the temporomandibular joint with pedicled temporalis muscle flaps. In: *Modern practice in orthognathic and reconstructive surgery.* Bell WH, Ed. Philadelphia, USA: Saunders, 1992: 733.

12 C.

The wider and higher the defect the greater the likelihood that a free flap will be required for reconstruction. The wider and higher the defect the greater the likelihood that a free flap will be needed. A Weber-Fergusson incision may be used for access. Involvement of the orbital floor would normally necessitate an exenteration for adequate tumour clearance. A free flap is indeed indicated in the wide and high defects and a DCIA flap allows for dental rehabilitation.

13 E.

Location on the buccal mucosa (as opposed to the floor of the mouth or tongue). The risk factors for malignant transformation include all those mentioned except the buccal mucosa. The floor of the mouth and tongue are high risk. Additional high-risk factors include the presence of epithelial dysplasia as well as non-homogeneous leukoplakia (combined red and white lesions). Mimics of leukoplakia include Candidiasis, discoid lupus, lichen planus, papillary hyperplasia secondary to ill-fitting dentures and white sponge naevi.

References
1.   Gnepp DR. *Diagnostic surgical pathology of the head and neck*, 2nd ed. Saunders-Elsevier, 2009: 9.

14 A.

Improper intra-operative seating of the condyles in the glenoid fossae.

References
1.   Mason ME, Schendel SA. Revision orthognathic surgery. In: *Maxillofacial surgery.* Booth PW, Schendel SA, Hausamen JE, Eds. New York, USA: Churchill Livingstone, 1999: 1321-34.

2.   McCarthy JG, Kawamoto HK, Grayson BH, Colen SR, Coccaro PJ. Surgery of the jaws. In: *Plastic surgery.* McCarthy JG, Ed. Philadelphia, USA: Saunders, 1990: 1188-474.

15 A.

Removal of all plates and immediate application of intermaxillary fixation.

References

1.   Jacques B, Richter M, Arza A. Treatment of mandibular fractures with rigid osteosynthesis: using the AO system. *J Oral Maxillofac Surg* 1997; 55(12): 1402-6.

2.   Koury ME, Perrott DH, Kaban LBN. The use of rigid internal fixation in mandibular fractures complicated by osteomyelitis. *J Oral Maxillofac Surg* 1994; 52(11): 1114-9.

16   D.

Neurotized free muscle transfer using innervation from cross-face grafts.

References

1.   Bove A, Chiarini S, D'Andrea V, Di Matteo FM, Lanzi G, De Antoni E. Facial nerve palsy: which flap? Microsurgical, anatomical, and functional considerations. *Microsurgery* 1998; 18(4): 286-9.

2.   Snyder MC, Johnson PJ, Moore GF, Ogren FP. Early versus late gold weight implantation for rehabilitation of the paralyzed eyelid. *Laryngoscope* 2001; 111(12): 2109-13.

3.   Wei W, Zuoliang Q, Xioaxi L, Jiasheng D, Chuan Y, Hussain K, Hongtai H, Gontur S, Li Z, Hua M, Tisheng C. Free split and segmental latissimus dorsi muscle transfer in one stage for facial reanimation. *Plast Reconstr Surg* 1999; 103(2): 473-80.

17   B and C.

Neurofibromata and *keloids*.

18   E.

Separation of the superior auricle from the temporal skin with placement of a retro-auricular skin graft.

References

1.   Furnas D. The correction of prominent ears by concha-mastoid sutures. *Plast Reconstr Surg* 1968; 42(3): 189-94.

2.   Leber D. Ear reconstruction. In: *Textbook of plastic, maxillofacial and reconstruction surgery*, 2nd ed. Georgiade GS, Riefkohl R, Levin LS, Eds. Baltimore, USA: Williams & Wilkins, 1996: 496.
3.   Mustardé J. The correction of prominent ears using mattress sutures. *Br J Plast Surg* 1963; 16: 170.

19 A.

A Bjork flap is an inferiorly-based U-shaped flap of anterior tracheal wall. Entering the trachea above the first cartilaginous ring would lead to vocal cord damage. The rings are below the cricoid cartilage. The parathyroids are not usually seen during the procedure, and there are blood vessels and the isthmus of the thyroid that cross the midline.

20 C.

Topical immunosuppressives have no role in its treatment. This statement is incorrect. Acute rejection is mediated by T-lymphocytes. There is also a high correlation between the clinical and histopathological findings of acute rejection. Acute rejection in the early stages is characterised by perivascular infiltration of lymphocytes in the upper and mid dermis. Early diagnosis and immunosuppressive adjustment result in high reversibility of acute rejection episodes. Topical drugs (tacrolimus, steroids or both) in combination with systemic immunosuppressives have been used successfully in the treatment of acute rejection in previous composite tissue transplantations.

21 D.

Repositioning/repair of the levator aponeurosis. Levator procedures require reasonable contractility of the levator muscle with fair to good levator function (>5mm) to elevate the lid. Dehiscence of the levator aponeurosis causes the most common type of ptosis. It is almost always an acquired condition, and its repair the commonest levator procedure undertaken. The indication is for circumstances where the aponeurosis has stretched (age-related) or has dehisced from the tarsal plate (trauma).

References

1.	Jelks GW, Smith BC. Reconstruction of the eyelids and associated structures. In: *Plastic surgery.* McCarthy JG, Ed. Philadelphia, USA: Saunders, 1990; 2: 1671-784.
2.	McCord CD Jr. The evaluation and management of the patient with ptosis. *Clin Plastic Surg* 1988; 15(2): 169-84.
3.	McCord CD, Codner MA. *Eyelid and periorbital surgery.* St Louis, USA: Quality Medical Publishing Inc., 2008: 406-59.

22 B.

19mm.

23 C.

10-70%. Based on extrapolations from clinical hand transplantations and also solid organ transplantation, the risk of acute rejection in facial transplantation is estimated to be between 10-70%. Almost all of these rejection episodes have been reversible, due to early diagnosis with visual inspection and adjustment in the maintenance immunosuppressive regimen and topical therapy.

24 A.

Is capable of identifying all enlarged nodes greater than 4-5mm in diameter.

25 B.

Soutar described the use of the radial forearm flap in oral cavity reconstruction. An approximate 10cm section of radius can also be taken, but it is advised that this is taken in a scaphoid shape and the radius plated to avoid fracture. Mandibular osteotomy should be undertaken more mesially to avoid alveolar nerve damage.

26   A and E.

Antitragus and *lobule*.

References

1.   Brent B. Reconstruction of auricle. In: *Plastic surgery*. McCarthy JG, Ed. Philadelphia, USA: Saunders Co, 1990: 3: 2094.

27   D.

Hypertrophic/keloid scar. The glassy collagen of keloids is distinctive, as is the tram-track pattern of positive smooth muscle actin on immunohistochemistry. Hypertrophic scars may also contain scattered S-100 protein positive cells representing Langerhans cells and proliferating nerve twigs. Desmin is usually negative. Readers should note that S-100 positivity is found in numerous cell types including nerves and Langerhans cells amongst others. It is not diagnostic of melanoma in isolation.

References

1.   Gnepp DR. *Diagnostic surgical pathology of the head and neck*, 2nd ed. Saunders-Elsevier, 2009: 647.

28   A.

Nasal polyps have a 2% malignant potential.

29   D.

A and C. The paramedian forehead flap receives blood supply from an extensive plexus of vessels around the medial brow area, which consists of the supratrochlear vessels as well as the angular branch interconnecting both the supraperiosteal and subperiosteal planes.

30 D.

Should leave the donor site open and allow healing by secondary intention.

31 A.

10%.

32 A and E.

Newborn infants and *relapsing polychondritis*.

33 E.

Spinal accessory nerve. The spinal accessory nerve is not in the left supraclavicular triangle of the neck. It runs mostly in the occipital/posterior triangle. The supraclavicular triangle is bounded by the inferior belly of omohyoid, the sternocleidomastoid (SCM), and the clavicle. The floor of the triangle is formed by the scalene muscles.

34 C.

Management is best delivered in a multidisciplinary setting.

35 C.

Zooming in to most magnification and focusing till the picture is sharp. Zooming to highest magnification and focusing till sharp will give the correct setting at the least depth of field. This will result in perfect sharpness at all lower magnifications up to the highest magnification at which the microscope was set.

36 B and D.

Is approximately 68mm long and *is larger than the female ear.* Ear size increases with age, especially the circumference as per the equation:

Ear circumference = 88.1 + (0.51 × subject's age).

References

1. Tan R, Osman V, Tan G. Ear size as a predictor of chronological age. *Archives of Gerontology and Geriatrics* 1997; 25(2): 187-91.

37 C.

Make sure there is no intimal damage in either vessel. The only real issue is to have good flow with undamaged intima and no debris inside the vessel or at the anastomotic site in a standard case with no other associated blood clotting or trauma issues.

38 C and E.

Chondrodermatitis and *gouty tophus.*

39 C.

Adult - thyroglossal duct cyst - most frequent. This is incorrect. The commonest cystic lesion of the head and neck in adults is metastatic cystic carcinoma. The others are correctly attributed.

References

1. Gnepp DR. *Diagnostic surgical pathology of the head and neck*, 2nd ed. Saunders-Elsevier, 2009: 841.

40 A.

The muscles are composed of four layers.

41 E.

Cheek flap. The Indian rhinoplasty uses forehead skin as did the local practitioners but Sushruta describes what we would now call a cheek advancement flap.

42 A and C.

Boys and *on the right.*

43 A.

Omohyoid originates from the upper border of the scapula and raises the hyoid bone. A is false. Omohyoid originates from the upper border of the scapula and has two separate insertions via the intermediate tendon onto the clavicle and first rib, and the hyoid bone lateral to the sternohyoid muscle. The blood supply to omohyoid is via the inferior thyroid artery. The two functions of omohyoid are to depress the hyoid and to tense the deep cervical fascia.

To describe the lymph nodes of the neck for neck dissection, the neck is divided into six areas called levels. The levels are identified by Roman numerals, increasing towards the chest. A further Level VII to denote lymph node groups in the superior mediastinum is no longer used. Instead, lymph nodes in other non-neck regions are referred to by the name of their specific nodal groups.

III includes lymph nodes of the middle jugular group. This level is bounded by the inferior border of the hyoid (superiorly) and the inferior border of the cricoid (inferiorly), the posterior border of the sternohyoid (anteriorly) and the posterior border of the SCM (posteriorly).

Level V includes the posterior compartment lymph nodes. This compartment is bounded by the clavicle (inferiorly), the anterior border of trapezius (posteriorly), and the posterior border of the SCM (anteriorly). It is divided into sublevels VA (lying above a transverse plane marking the inferior border of the anterior cricoid arch) and VB (below the aforementioned plane).

Bocca popularised the functional neck dissection in the 1960s, and is often referred to as the originator of the technique; however, it appears that other surgeons were performing such dissections before him.

References

1.   Ferlito A, Rinaldo A. Osvaldo Suárez: often-forgotten father of functional neck dissection (in the non-Spanish-speaking literature). *Laryngoscope* 2004; 114(7): 1177-8.

2.   Bocca E. Supraglottic laryngectomy and functional neck dissection. *J Laryngol Otol* 1966; 80(8): 831-8.

44 D.

Marginal mandibulectomy. A tumour of this size with nodal spread needs segmental excision and definitive reconstruction with postoperative radiotherapy. Central tumours and those involving or crossing the midline require bilateral neck dissection.

45 D.

Muller's muscle may be dysfunctional.

46 B.

Is likely to be a metastasis. Whilst there is undoubted geographical and demographic difference in tumour types, this is the best answer amongst the choices given, and is usually a metastatic SCC. In Australia, metastasis from squamous carcinoma or melanoma accounts for up to

75% of parotid malignancy. The commonest benign tumour is pleomorphic adenoma (the treatment for which has evolved from superficial parotidectomy to wide local excision). The commonest primary malignant tumour in most series is muco-epidermoid carcinoma, although some texts mistakenly suggest carcinoma ex-pleomorphic adenoma is the commonest malignancy. Gustatory sweating is Frey's syndrome and is a complication of parotidectomy. Fine needle aspiration is a good diagnostic modality for parotid tumours.

References

1.   Gnepp DR. *Diagnostic surgical pathology of the head and neck*, 2nd ed. Saunders-Elsevier, 2009: 413-562.

47 B.

Facial artery.

48 A.

McFee described the classical 'Y' incision used for neck dissection. A is false. Neck incisions for neck dissection include: Lahey (1940), Martin (1951), Slaughter (1955), Schobinger (1957), Conley (1966), McFee (1960) and Ariyan (1980). The 'Y' incisions provide excellent exposure but necrosis of the tips may result and expose the vascular structures. McFee described two transverse incisions to approach neck nodes in 1960. The bipedicled McFee has a better blood supply but more tedious exposure. The hockey stick incision (Ariyan) is performed from mastoid to shoulder, behind the anterior border of the trapezius muscle and extending medially below the clavicle. The apron flap extends from mastoid to mastoid passing along the posterior border of the SCM to the midline, 2-3 fingerbreadths above the sternal notch.

The TNM system (Table 1) is based on clinical evaluation of the patient. Staging is used to compare the results of different treatments and between institutions, to estimate prognosis in terms of tumour control and patient survival, to plan treatment and to influence the choice of therapy.

Table 1. Classification for primary tumour of the larynx.

Tx   Primary cannot be assessed.
T0   No evidence of primary.
Tis   Carcinoma *in situ.*
Supraglottis:
T1   Tumour limited to one subsite of supraglottis or glottis with normal vocal cord mobility.
T2   Tumour invades more than one subsite of supraglottis with normal vocal cord mobility.
T3   Tumour limited to the larynx with vocal cord fixation or invades postcricoid area, medial wall of pyriform sinus, or pre-epiglottic tissues.
T4   Tumour invades through thyroid cartilage or extends to other tissues beyond the larynx, e.g. to oropharynx, soft tissues of the neck.
Glottis:
T1   Tumour limited to vocal cord(s) (may involve anterior or posterior commissures) with normal mobility.
T2   Tumour extends to supraglottis or subglottis, or with impaired vocal cord mobility.
T3   Tumour limited to the larynx with vocal cord fixation.
T4   Tumour invades through thyroid cartilage or extends to other tissues beyond the larynx, e.g. to oropharynx or soft tissues of the neck.
Subglottis:
T1   Tumour limited to the subglottis.
T2   Tumour extends to vocal cord(s) with normal or impaired mobility.
T3   Tumour limited to the larynx with vocal cord fixation.
T4   Tumour invades through cricoid or thyroid cartilage or extends to other tissues beyond the larynx, e.g. to oropharynx or soft tissues of the neck.

N0   No regional node involvement.
N1   Ipsilateral regional nodes less than 3cm.
N2   Single ipsilateral node 3-6cm or multiple ipsilateral nodes less than 6cm; or bilateral or contralateral nodes, not greater than 6cm.
N3   Massive ipsilateral nodes or contralateral nodes (greater than 6cm).

M0   No evidence of distant metastases.
M1   Metastases beyond the cervical lymph nodes.

Stage 0	Tis N0 M0
Stage I	T1 N0 M0
Stage II	T2 N0 M0
Stage III	T3 N0 M0
	T1 N1 M0
	T2 N1 M0
	T3 N1 M0
Stage IV	T4 N0/N1 M0
	Any T, N2/N3 M0
	Any T, any N, M1

References

1.   McFee WF. Transverse incisions for neck dissection. *Ann Surg* 1960; 151(2): 279-84.

2.   Crile G. Excision of cancer of the head and neck. *J Am Med Assoc* 1906; 47: 1780-6.

49 E.

There have been no recorded mortalities so far following face transplantation. E is false. At least two of the initial face transplant recipients has died. One was linked to lack of patient compliance with immunotherapy, and the other was reportedly due to a cardiac event whilst undergoing revisional surgery.

50 D.

Lies deep to the SMAS layer. The parotid gland contains almost exclusively serous cells although a few mucous acini are found in the tail of the parotid close to the submandibular gland. The parotid duct opens into the oral cavity opposite the second maxillary molar tooth.

51 A.

The pathophysiology of mandibular invasion from an oral cancer alters after radiotherapy.

52 C.

Pfeiffer's syndrome. This is not a cause of facial palsy. The causes of facial palsy can be broadly divided into intracranial, intratemporal and extratemporal. Several patterns of facial nerve dysfunction point to a non-idiopathic cause: simultaneous bilateral facial palsy (Guillain-Barré syndrome, sarcoidosis, pseudobulbar palsy, syphilis, leukaemia, trauma, Wegener's granulomatosis), unilateral facial weakness slowly progressing beyond 3 weeks (cholesteatoma, facial nerve neuroma, metastatic carcinoma, adenoid cystic carcinoma), slowly progressive unilateral facial weakness associated with facial hyperkinesis (facial nerve neuroma), no return of facial nerve function within 6 months after abrupt onset of palsy (facial nerve neuroma, adenoid cystic carcinoma, basal cell carcinoma), ipsilateral lateral rectus palsy, and recurrent unilateral facial palsy (facial nerve neuroma, adenoid cystic carcinoma, meningioma).

Several viruses have been implicated including *Varicella zoster*, *Herpes simplex* and Epstein-Barr. Facial paralysis occurs in 11% of patients with Lyme disease; in 30% of cases, the paralysis is bilateral. AIDS is also an increasingly common cause of bilateral involvement.

Pfeiffer's syndrome is not associated with facial nerve palsy. This syndrome is characterised by: craniosynostosis (most often of the coronal and lambdoid), and midfacial hypoplasia with receded cheekbones or exophthalmos. Ocular proptosis and hypertelorism, broad thumbs and big toes are other features. The mental capacity of Pfeiffer patients is usually in the normal range.

53 D.

May lead to a hoarse voice postoperatively.

54 B.

Patients may be able to speak and swallow after an appropriate reconstruction.

55 D.

According to Mathes and Nahai, the fibula bone, like the pectoralis muscle, has a Type V vascular pattern. The length of the pedicle to the fibula flap depends on the site of the proximal osteotomy rather than the length of the peroneal vessels from their origin to the tibial side of the bone. Along the fibula, the pedicle must be dissected in a subperiosteal plane to preserve bone vascularity. Arteria peronea magna is an absolute contraindication to free fibula flap harvest due to the risk of foot devascularisation. The double-barrelled fibula flap configuration was first described by Yoo *et al* [1]; Jupiter *et al* [2] published their report some 5 years later. The fibula bone has a Mathes and Nahai Type V pattern of circulation; their classification is not limited to muscles and muscle-containing flaps. Unicortical screw fixation of the osteotomised free fibula is recommended over bicortical fixation to safeguard the periosteal blood supply to the bone.

References

1.   Yoo MC, *et al*. Free vascularized fibular graft using microsurgical technique. *J Korean Orthop Assoc* 1982; 17: 403.

2.   Jupiter JB, Bour CJ, May JW. The reconstruction of defects in the femoral shaft with vascularized transfers of fibular bone. *J Bone Joint Surg [Am]* 1987; 69: 365-74.

Section 7 questions

Cutaneous malignancy and sarcoma

1   Which of these is not a predisposing factor to the development of melanoma?

A.   Giant congenital melanocytic naevus.
B.   Familial dysplastic naevus syndrome.
C.   Pseudoxanthoma elasticum.
D.   >50 acquired melanocytic naevi.
E.   Xeroderma pigmentosum.

2   With regards to cutaneous 'horns':

A.   These should never be treated with surgery.
B.   They are always benign.
C.   They often arise from basal cell carcinomata.
D.   They always arise from squamous carcinomata.
E.   None of the above.

3   The most common cancer of the ear is:

A.   Malignant melanoma.
B.   Basal cell carcinoma (BCC).
C.   Squamous cell carcinoma (SCC).
D.   Metastatic deposits.
E.   Adnexal tumour.

4 Which is not a tumour known to commonly arise from a sebaceous (organoid) naevus?

A. BCC.
B. Tricholemmoma.
C. Mycosis fungoides.
D. SCC.
E. Syringocystadenoma papilliferum.

5 Which statement is incorrect about Merkel cell tumour?

A. Usually occurs in the head and neck.
B. Is an adenocarcinoma of neuroendocrine origin.
C. Has a high recurrence rate.
D. Postoperative radiotherapy is recommended.
E. Is sometimes benign.

6 The following are histopathological terms correctly matched with their meanings:

A. Parakeratosis: where nucleated cells are found in the superficial epidermis.
B. Maturation: where naevocellular naevi become more superficially cited in the epidermis.
C. Peripheral pallisading: a feature of poorly differentiated squamous carcinoma.
D. Erythroplakia - red lesions of the oral mucosa.
E. Leukoplakia - white lesions of the oral mucosa.

7 Features of Gorlin's syndrome do not include:

A. Medulloblastoma.
B. Multiple BCC.
C. Keratocyst of the jaw.

D.   Bifid ribs.
E.   Hypospadias.

8   Which of the following is incorrect about cutaneous squamous cell carcinoma?

A.   It is more common than BCC.
B.   It has a higher metastatic rate than BCC.
C.   It has an increased incidence in the immunosuppressed.
D.   SCC of the lip has a higher metastatic rate to lymph nodes.
E.   The role of sentinel node biopsy has been established.

9   Which of the following statements is correct?

A.   The hamstring muscles include semimembranosus, semitendinosus and gracilis.
B.   The dominant action of biceps femoris is to flex the hip joint.
C.   The sciatic nerve is accessible in the angle between the lower border of gluteus maximus and the medial border of the long head of biceps femoris.
D.   All but one of the motor branches of the sciatic nerve arises from its medial side, making the lateral side the safest side to dissect along.
E.   None of the above is true.

10   For a melanoma of the same depth which of the following has a worse prognosis?

A.   Superficial spreading melanoma.
B.   Nodular melanoma.
C.   Lentigo maligna melanoma.
D.   Acral lentiginous melanoma.
E.   None of the above.

11 With regard to the adductor compartment of the thigh, which of the following is not true?

A. The femoral artery and profunda femoris artery are separated by adductor longus at the level of the middle of the thigh.
B. Adductor magnus inserts on the medial border of the tibial plateau.
C. The femoral artery becomes the politeal artery at the adductor hiatus in adductor magnus.
D. Adductor magnus arises from both the posterior and anterior aspects of the ischium.
E. Adductor brevis arises from the inferior ramus of the pubis.

12 With regards to actinic keratoses, which is false?

A. Typical histologic features include a background of elastosis.
B. They can be treated using topical 5-fluorouracil.
C. They can be treated using topical diclofenac.
D. They can be treated using cryotherapy.
E. They should always be treated with wide local excision.

13 Which of the following is not true in relation to the femoral triangle?

A. The inguinal ligament forms the base.
B. The lateral border of adductor longus forms the medial side.
C. The medial border of tensor fascia lata forms the lateral side.
D. The femoral artery and vein lie in front of the fascia covering ilio-psoas and the femoral nerve lies behind it.
E. At the apex, four vessels and two nerves pass into the adductor canal of Hunter.

14 When biopsying melanoma:

A. Incision biopsy is absolutely contraindicated.
B. Punch biopsy is an absolute contraindication.

C. Incisional biopsy worsens the prognosis.
D. A suspicious subungual lesion should be biopsied with a punch or incisional technique.
E. None of the above.

15 The following predispose to mesenchymal neoplasia except:

A. Tuberous sclerosis.
B. HIV.
C. Familial lipomatosis.
D. Megavoltage irradiation.
E. Arthrogryphosis congenita multiplex.

16 Which of the following is not correct with respect to the axilla?

A. The axilla has three muscular walls and one bony wall.
B. The posterior wall comprises latissimus dorsi, teres major and subscapularis.
C. The medial wall is serratus anterior.
D. The axillary artery and vein pass in front of the tendon of pectoralis minor as it passes superiorly to insert into the coracoid process.
E. The anterior border is defined by pectoralis major, pectoralis minor and subclavius.

17 Regarding melanoma:

A. Nodular histological types have no radial growth phase.
B. Acral melanomas account for 30% of lesions.
C. Lentigo maligna is the commonest subtype.
D. Superficial spreading melanoma is common on the palms of the hand.
E. Desmoplastic subtypes are negative for the S100 histological marker.

18 From the following statements regarding the prognosis for patients with primary cutaneous malignant melanoma, which is incorrect?

A. In general, the prognosis for women is significantly better than for men.

B. Older patients have a worse prognosis than younger patients.

C. Ulceration is a poor prognostic factor.

D. The total vertical height (Breslow thickness) is the single most important prognostic variable for stage I and II melanoma.

E. Five-year survival for a patient with a melanoma of Breslow thickness of 4mm without evidence of metastases is approximately 15%.

19 The following are specific risk factors for melanoma except:

A. More than 50 ordinary moles.

B. A single dysplastic naevus.

C. Age over 50.

D. Male sex.

E. Blue eyes.

20 The following is false concerning photodynamic therapy (PDT):

A. Evidence of efficacy of this procedure for the treatment of BCC, Bowen's disease and actinic (solar) keratosis is adequate to support its use for these conditions, provided that the normal arrangements are in place for consent, audit and clinical governance.

B. There is early evidence that PDT in combination with CO_2 laser may be successfully used in the treatment of nodular basal carcinomas.

C.   It is a good choice for treatment of low-risk SCCs, but only those of the well-differentiated subtype.
D.   PDT is not a good choice for high-risk lesions such as those of the medial canthus.
E.   PDT is not a good option for the treatment of morpheic BCC.

21 Which of the following prognostic features of melanoma is not included in the AJCC staging system?

A.   Ulceration.
B.   Mitotic rate.
C.   Clarke's level of invasion.
D.   Micrometastasis to lymph nodes.
E.   Lactate dehydrogenase (LDH).

22 Which of the following are risk factors for cutaneous melanoma?

A.   Melasma.
B.   Childhood UV exposure.
C.   Fitzpatrick Type 5 skin.
D.   Previous radiotherapy.
E.   Fifteen pre-existing benign naevi.

23 Dysplastic naevus syndrome is characterised by:

A.   X-linked recessive genetic inheritance.
B.   >100 naevi with at least one clinically atypical naevus.
C.   50% risk of developing melanoma.
D.   Naevi present at birth.
E.   Causation associated with solarium tanning beds.

24 With respect to sentinel lymph node biopsy in melanoma, which is the best answer?

A. It provides prognostic information.
B. It improves staging.
C. It is used to guide adjuvant therapy.
D. A positive result mandates completion lymph node dissection (CLND).
E. All of the above.

25 In relation to axillary lymphadenectomy:

A. The axillary vein lies lateral to the axillary artery.
B. The average number of lymph nodes in each axilla is between 70 and 80.
C. Tributaries of the axillary vein should all be divided.
D. The thoracodorsal artery must be sacrificed to allow clearance of level 3 nodes.
E. Division of pectoralis minor is commonly undertaken for improved access.

26 Which of these immunohistochemistry markers is incorrectly matched with its skin pathology?

A. Cytokeratin and SCC.
B. S100 and melanoma.
C. CD34 and dermatofibroma sarcoma protuberans.
D. HMB45 and BCC.
E. CD31 and angiosarcoma.

27 Melanomas arise from:

A. Superficial keratinocytes.
B. Apocrine sweat glands.
C. Neural crest cells.
D. Hair follicles.
E. Ectopic mucosa.

28 The following is false concerning basal cell carcinomas:

A. Nodular lesions grow downward deep into the dermis as cords and islands of variably basophilic cells with hyperchromatic nuclei, embedded in a mucinous matrix and are often surrounded by fibroblasts and lymphocytes.
B. Perivascular and perineural invasion are features associated with more aggressive tumours.
C. The reported incomplete excision rate of BCCs is approximately 7%.
D. The estimation of surgical excision margins is often inaccurate.
E. Radiotherapy is effective in the treatment of primary BCC, surgically recurrent BCC, radio-recurrent BCC and as adjuvant therapy, and is thought to be the treatment of choice for high-risk disease in patients who are unwilling or unable to tolerate surgery.

29 Which of the following are predisposing risk factors for the development of skin cancer?

A. Sebaceous naevus of Jadassohn.
B. Gorlin's syndrome.
C. Xeroderma pigmentosa.
D. Albinism.
E. All of the above.

30 The following best describes a 1.1mm ulcerated melanoma with micrometastasis in a sentinel lymph node:

A.   T2bN1b.
B.   Stage 3B.
C.   Stage 4.
D.   Stage 2C.
E.   None of the above.

31 With respect to basal cell carcinoma:

A.   It occurs most commonly on the arms and legs.
B.   It is not related to sun exposure.
C.   There is a higher recurrence rate with the infiltrative subtype.
D.   Histology classically shows pagetoid spread in the epidermis.
E.   It has a 2% metastasis rate.

32 The following best describes a 3.1mm non-ulcerated melanoma with no nodal or distant metastasis:

A.   T3aN0M0.
B.   Stage 4.
C.   Stage 3A.
D.   Stage 2C.
E.   Stage 2B.

33 Which of the following skin pathologies and their classic histologic features are correctly matched?

A.   Dermatofibroma sarcoma protuberans and basophilic cells with peripheral pallisading.
B.   Melanoma and eosinophilic cells with keratin production.
C.   BCC and storeiform arrangement of fibroblasts.

D. Merkel cell carcinoma (MCC) and small basophilic neuroendocrine cells.
E. None of the above.

34 The following best describes a 3.5mm ulcerated melanoma with no nodal or distant metastasis:

A. T3bN1M0.
B. Stage 4.
C. Stage 3A.
D. Stage 2C.
E. Stage 2B.

35 A patient with a 1cm diameter SCC of the lower lip vermillion:

A. Will not develop cervical node metastases.
B. Should undergo bilateral prophylactic neck dissection.
C. Should be treated with an upper lip Abbé flap.
D. Can be preferentially treated with photodynamic therapy with or without CO_2 laser.
E. Requires excision with a minimum 4mm margin.

36 Which of the following statements regarding sentinel lymph node biopsy in melanoma is false?

A. It is the best prognostic indicator for overall survival.
B. It allows improved staging.
C. It allows identification of patients to enter clinical trials.
D. It leads to a definite increase in overall survival.
E. There is a probable increase in disease-free survival.

37 The following is true regarding melanoma:

A.   A margin of 3cm must be taken for a 2.2mm lesion.
B.   A better prognosis exists for a stage IIIA melanoma than for a IIC melanoma at 5 years.
C.   Back lesions have the best prognosis.
D.   Suspicious lesions should be best sampled with a punch biopsy forcep.
E.   It never metastasizes to the thyroid.

38 The following is true regarding melanoma:

A.   A patient with a 0.7mm lesion has at least a 10% risk of death by 10 years.
B.   MM250 is the most sensitive immunohistological marker.
C.   HNB75 is the most sensitive immunohistological marker.
D.   *In situ* lesions have a Breslow thickness less than 0.15mm.
E.   *In situ* melanomas are the same lesions as solar lentigo in all but name.

39 The following is true regarding melanoma:

A.   It is more common in women.
B.   Has a better prognosis in patients with black skin.
C.   A Spitz naevus is synonymous with juvenile melanoma.
D.   Is more common in brunettes than blondes.
E.   There is a 50% lifetime risk in giant hairy naevi.

40 The following is true regarding melanoma:

A.   Nodular is the commonest subtype.
B.   Is most commonly found on the scalp of men and the backs of women.
C.   Is most commonly found on the legs of men and the backs of women.

D.   It has an 88% 10-year survival if <1mm Breslow thickness.
E.   *In situ* melanoma has a 95% 10-year survival.

41 In relation to Bowen's disease of skin:

A.   It must be excised with 1cm margins.
B.   Can be treated successfully with photodynamic therapy.
C.   Most often occurs on the scalp of men.
D.   Is a precursor of squamous carcinoma *in situ*.
E.   Most commonly affects the nipple.

42 In relation to basal cell carcinoma:

A.   Metastasis never occurs.
B.   Is the most commonly occuring cancer of the lower lip.
C.   A 4mm margin on the face gives a cure rate of greater than 90%.
D.   Are never pigmented.
E.   Are familial in Gordon's syndrome.

Section 7 answers

Cutaneous malignancy and sarcoma

1 C.

Pseudoxanthoma elasticum. Pseudoxanthoma elasticum is not a predisposing factor to the development of melanoma. It is a genetic disorder of elastic tissue involving skin, eyes and the cardiovascular system with no malignant potential. All the others can predispose to the development of melanoma. Acquired melanocytic naevi (MN) in Caucasian populations are important markers for the risk of melanoma development. The total number of MN on the whole body is the most important independent risk factor for melanoma and the risk of melanoma development increases almost linearly with rising numbers of MN (the average person has 20-40 acquired naevi).

2 E.

None of the above. Cutaneous horns may originate from well-differentiated squamous carcinomata (5-15%), but the majority are benign. They may warrant excision both on symptomatic grounds and to exclude malignancy.

3 C.

Squamous cell carcinoma (SCC).

4 C.

Mycosis fungoides. This is not a tumour known to commonly arise from a sebaceous naevus. BCC is the most common malignant tumour, but benign tumours such as tricholemmoma, trichoblastoma and syringocystadenoma are much more common. Mycosis fungoides is a cutaneous T-cell lymphoma and is unrelated. Older series suggested malignant potential to be 10-15%, but more recent series suggest this rate is much lower. The tumours arise in adolescence or early adult life but can occur in children under 5 years.

5 E.

Is sometimes benign. This statement is incorrect; Merkel cell tumours are always malignant. They usually occur in the head and neck and they are an adenocarcinoma of neuroendocrine origin. Due to their high recurrence rates and radiosensitivity, postoperative radiotherapy is recommended.

6 A.

Parakeratosis: where nucleated cells are found in the superficial epidermis. Parakeratosis is where nuclei of keratinocytes persist as they rise into the horny layer of the skin; it occurs normally in the epithelium of mucous membranes. When it occurs on the external skin it constitutes a lesion. Maturation is where naevus cells migrate into the dermis. Peripheral pallisading is classically seen in basal carcinoma and occasionally 'basi-squamous' carcinoma (a controversial diagnosis). Neither erythroplakia nor leukoplakia are histopathological terms - they denote clinical appearances, although they are both correctly defined.

7 E.

Hypospadias. All the others are features of Gorlin's syndrome except hypospadias. Additional features include macrocephaly, distinct facial features, frontal bossing, palmar and plantar skin pits, cleft lip and palate, and ectopic calcification, e.g. falx cerebri.

8 A.

It is more common than BCC. A is incorrect. BCC is approximately 2.5 times more common than SCC.

9 D.

All but one of the motor branches of the sciatic nerve arises from its medial side, making the lateral side the safest side to dissect along. The only motor branch to arise from the lateral border of the sciatic nerve is the branch to the short head of biceps and so it is safest to dissect along the lateral side. The hamstrings are semimembranosus, semitendinosus and the long head of biceps femoris (only). They extend the hip and flex the knee. The sciatic nerve is deep in the angle between gluteus maximus and the lateral border of the long head of biceps. The short head of biceps is not considered part of the hamstrings because it does not arise from the ischium and has no action on the hip joint.

10 E.

None of the above. Depth is an independent risk factor.

11 B.

Adductor magnus inserts on the medial border of the tibial plateau. B is incorrect. The adductor magnus arises from both aspects of the ischium and inserts into the superior border of the medial condyle of the femur and also the gluteal tuberosity of the posterior femur. The hamstrings lie laterally to the adductor and insert into the tibia. The femoral artery and profunda femoris artery are separated by the medial border of adductor longus. The profunda lies on the anterior aspect of adductor brevis and posterior to vastus medialis at this point.

12 E.

They should always be treated with wide local excision. E is false. Actinic (solar) keratoses are premalignant lesions related to ultraviolet sun exposure and predispose particularly to SCC. Numerous topical treatments can be used successfully. Surgery is reserved for lesions suspicious of malignancy, for biopsy, or for especially symptomatic lesions that are keratotic. If excision is undertaken, the margins should be minimal and not wide to allow an accurate histopathological diagnosis prior to planning further treatment.

13 c.

The medial border of tensor fascia lata forms the lateral side. This statement is incorrect; the lateral border of the femoral canal is the sartorius muscle. While some authorities consider that the medial border of adductor longus forms the medial side, they are in the minority. At the apex, the femoral A&V, profunda femoris A&V, saphenous N. and N. to vastus medialis enter Hunter's canal. The femoral artery passes from the midpoint of the base of the triangle to the apex.

14 d.

A suspicious subungual lesion should be biopsied with a punch or incisional technique.

15 e.

Arthrogryphosis congenita multiplex. Anthrogryphosis is not associated with mesenchymal tumours - all the others are. HIV is associated with cutaneous (Kaposi) sarcoma. Tuberous sclerosis is associated with angiofibromas and hamartomas as well as lipomas.

References
1.   Gnepp DR. *Diagnostic surgical pathology of the head and neck*, 2nd ed. Saunders-Elsevier, 2009: 975-1068.

16 d.

The axillary artery and vein pass in front of the tendon of pectoralis minor as it passes superiorly to insert into the coracoid process. This statement is incorrect; the axillary artery and vein actually pass behind the tendon of pectoralis minor. The bony wall of the axilla is the inter-tubercular sulcus of the humerus and is concealed by biceps and coracobrachialis.

17 A.

Nodular histological types have no radial growth phase. The commonest subtype is superficial spreading melanoma (approximately 70%). Acral lentiginous melanomas are the most common subtype found on the palm of the hand, and acral melanomas account for less than 10% of lesions except in those with black skin where they may account for between 35-60% of lesions. Other subtypes include desmoplastic, amelanotic, and mucosal melanoma.

References
1.   Janis JE. *Essentials of plastic surgery.* St Louis, USA: Quality Medical Publishing Inc., 2007: 124-5.

18 E.

Five-year survival for a patient with a melanoma of Breslow thickness of 4mm without evidence of metastases is approximately 15%. This statement is incorrect. In a big published series the 5-year survival for a patient with a thick melanoma of 4mm Breslow thickness and no evidence of metastases is still greater than 50%. Female sex on its own is a good prognostic factor, probably because women tend to present with thinner lesions on the extremities - itself a good variable. The presence of ulceration significantly worsens prognosis. Older patients do less well but this is probably because they tend to present with thicker lesions. Breslow thickness is a better prognostic variable than Clark's level or tumour/skin thickness ratios.

References
1.   Balch CM, Buzaid AC, Soong SJ, Atkins MB, Cascinelli N, Coit DG, Fleming ID, Gershenwald JE, Houghton A Jr, Kirkwood JM, McMasters KM, Mihm MF, Morton DL, Reintgen DS, Ross MI, Sober A, Thompson JA, Thompson JF. Final version of the American Joint Committee on Cancer Staging system for cutaneous melanoma. *J Clin Oncol* 2001; 19(16): 3635-48.

19 E.

Blue eyes. Risk factors for melanoma include: UV light exposure, increased age, Fitzpatrick Type 1 and 2 skin, red hair, male sex (1:49 vs 1:72 lifetime risk men vs women), family history, atypical naevus syndromes, congenital naevi (small increased risk), greater than 50 typical moles, and lentigo maligna. A single dysplastic naevus has a 6-10% lifetime risk of malignant transformation.

References

1.   Janis JE. *Essentials of plastic surgery.* St Louis, USA: Quality Medical Publishing Inc., 2007: 122-3.

20 C.

It is a good choice for treatment of low-risk SCCs, but only those of the well-differentiated subtype. C is false. There is good evidence for efficacy of photodynamic therapy for the treatment of basal cell carcinoma (BCC), Bowen's disease and actinic (solar) keratosis and this evidence is adequate to support its use for these conditions provided that the normal arrangements are in place for consent, audit and clinical governance. Evidence is lacking in relation to SCC, and the chance of local recurrence and metastatic risk is too high. There is a good summary of indications and evidence for PDT in the UK NICE guidelines [1]. A study in 2007 reported that CO_2 laser and PDT appeared to play a synergistic role in the treatment of nodular BCCs. The cosmetic results were excellent and the mean recurrence-free follow-up was 18.1 months [2]. Photodynamic therapy should not generally be used on areas such as the medial canthus or used for the treatment of morpheic BCCs. The lack of histological confirmation of clearance and high risk of local recurrence in these situations preclude its widespread use with current evidence.

References

1.   http://www.nice.org.uk/guidance/IPG155/Guidance/pdf/English.
2.   Whitaker IS, Shokrollahi K, James W, Mishra A, Lohana P, Murison MC. Combined CO_2 laser with photodynamic therapy for the treatment of nodular basal cell carcinomas. *Ann Plast Surg* 2007; 59(5): 484-8.

21 B.

Mitotic rate. The American Joint Committee for Cancer staging system has undergone several revisions; however, it uses the TNM staging system. T (tumour) staging includes Clark's level and ulceration as prognostic factors. N (node) staging includes micro-metastases, and M (metastases) includes LDH as a prognostic factor. Mitotic rate is not used.

References

1.   Balch CM, Buzaid AC, Soong SJ, Atkins MB, Cascinelli N, Coit DG, Fleming ID, Gershenwald JE, Houghton A Jr, Kirkwood JM, McMasters KM, Mihm MF, Morton DL, Reintgen DS, Ross MI, Sober A, Thompson JA, Thompson JF. Final version of the American Joint Committee on Cancer Staging system for cutaneous melanoma. *J Clin Oncol* 2001; 19(16): 3635-48.

22 B.

Childhood UV exposure. Cutaneous melanoma has an increased risk with light hair colour, lower Fitzpatrick skin Type (1 and 2), and dysplastic naevi (no benign naevi). Radiotherapy is related to an increased risk of sarcomas. A history of blistering sunburn in childhood is a risk factor. Melasma (chloasma) is hormonal-related pigmentation of the skin commonly seen in women, especially during pregnancy and when taking hormone-replacement therapy or oral contraception. It does not have a risk of malignant transformation.

23 B.

>100 naevi with at least one clinically atypical naevus. Atypical moles can be inherited or sporadic. Formal genetic analysis has suggested an autosomal dominant mode of inheritance (not X-linked). The risk of developing malignant melanoma approaches 100%. Naevi begin to develop in childhood.

24 E.

All of the above. While there is still debate as to the role of sentinel lymph node biopsy in melanoma staging, the results of a sentinel node biopsy do provide prognostic and staging information. This information guides adjuvant therapy and certainly mandates completion nodal dissection, if nodal metastases are found.

25 E.

Division of pectoralis minor is commonly undertaken for improved access. The axillary vein is medial to the axillary artery and the axilla usually contains 20-30 nodes.

References

1.   Stone C, Ed. *The evidence for plastic surgery.* Shrewsbury, UK: tfm publishing Ltd, 2008.

26 D.

HMB45 and BCC. This is incorrect. Melan A, S100 and HMB45 are all markers for melanoma, while BCC markers are less specific and include EMA, CEA and bcl-2. The other markers are correctly attributed.

27 C.

Neural crest cells.

28 E.

Radiotherapy is effective in the treatment of primary BCC, surgically recurrent BCC, radio-recurrent BCC and as adjuvant therapy, and is thought to be the treatment of choice for high-risk disease in patients who are unwilling or unable to tolerate surgery. E is false. Nodular BCCs grow downward deep into the dermis as cords and islands of variably basophilic cells with hyperchromatic nuclei, embedded in a mucinous matrix and are often surrounded by fibroblasts and lymphocytes. Multifocal superficial BCCs originate in the epidermis and often extend over several square centimetres or more. Histological features of aggression include perivascular and perineural invasion [1]. In an audit of 1392 BCCs arising in 1165 patients, excised under the care of one surgeon in the 10 years from 1988 to 1997, 99 (7%) were reported histologically as incompletely excised [2]. In a study in 2003, surgeons of differing experience (n=19) marked excision margins of 2, 5 and 10mm around a standard circular lesion drawn on paper [3]. Use of surgical markers, rulers and loupe magnification were all permitted, with five attempts for each margin. The percentage error found was 35, 14 and 4% for the 2, 5 and 10mm margins, respectively (regardless of the grade of surgeon). Repetition of the experiment on volunteer skin demonstrated a percentage error of 45, 16 and 8% for 2, 5 and 10mm margins (significantly greater than the corresponding errors on paper, p<0.001 in all cases). Radiotherapy is NOT effective in the treatment of radio-recurrent BCC.

References

1.   Telfer NR, Colver GB, Morton CA; British Association of Dermatologists. Guidelines for the management of basal cell carcinoma. *Br J Dermatol* 2008; 1 59(1): 35-48.

2.   Griffiths RW. Audit of histologically incompletely excised basal cell carcinomas: recommendations for management by re-excision. *Br J Plast Surg* 1999; 52(1): 24-8.

3.   Lalla R, Brown TL, Griffiths RW. Where to draw the line: the error in marking surgical excision margins defined. *Br J Plast Surg* 2003; 56(6): 603-6.

4.   Kumar V, Abbas AK, Fausto N. *Robbins & Cotran pathologic basis of disease*, 7th ed. Philadelphia, USA: WB Saunders, 2004.

29 E.

All of the above. Sebaceous naevus of Jadassohn (organoid naevus) has a propensity to BCC development (amongst other benign and malignant tumours). Gorlin's syndrome (basal cell naevus syndrome) is also associated with BCCs. Albinism is associated with an increased risk of both SCC and BCC. Xeroderma pigmentosa is associated with a significantly increased risk of BCC, SCC and melanoma.

30 B.

Stage 3B. The AJCC classification for melanoma is widely published.

References

1. Balch CM, Buzaid AC, Soong SJ, Atkins MB, Cascinelli N, Coit DG, Fleming ID, Gershenwald JE, Houghton A Jr, Kirkwood JM, McMasters KM, Mihm MF, Morton DL, Reintgen DS, Ross MI, Sober A, Thompson JA, Thompson JF. Final version of the American Joint Committee on Cancer Staging system for cutaneous melanoma. *J Clin Oncol* 2001; 19(16): 3635-48.

31 C.

There is a higher recurrence rate with the infiltrative subtype. Recurrence is greatest in the infiltrative subtype. Morpheaform (sclerosing) subtype is also associated with a high recurrence rate. Metastases are limited to case reports/small case series.

32 A.

T3aN0M0 (Stage IIA). The AJCC classification for melanoma is widely reproduced.

References

1. Balch CM, Buzaid AC, Soong SJ, Atkins MB, Cascinelli N, Coit DG, Fleming ID, Gershenwald JE, Houghton A Jr, Kirkwood JM, McMasters KM, Mihm MF, Morton DL, Reintgen DS, Ross MI, Sober A, Thompson JA, Thompson JF. Final version of the American Joint Committee on Cancer Staging system for cutaneous melanoma. *J Clin Oncol* 2001; 19(16): 3635-48.

33 D.

Merkel cell carcinoma (MCC) and small basophilic neuroendocrine cells. Basophilic cells with peripheral pallisading is a feature of nodular BCC. Keratin production is rare in melanoma, but common in SCC, and storeiform arrangement of fibroblasts is associated with dermatofibroma sarcoma protuberans.

34 E.

Stage 2B. The AJCC classification for melanoma is widely published.

References

1. Balch CM, Buzaid AC, Soong SJ, Atkins MB, Cascinelli N, Coit DG, Fleming ID, Gershenwald JE, Houghton A Jr, Kirkwood JM, McMasters KM, Mihm MF, Morton DL, Reintgen DS, Ross MI, Sober A, Thompson JA, Thompson JF. Final version of the American Joint Committee on Cancer Staging system for cutaneous melanoma. *J Clin Oncol* 2001; 19(16): 3635-48.

35 E.

Requires excision with a minimum 4mm margin. Guidelines published by Motley *et al* recommend 4mm margins for low-risk lesions and 6mm margins for high-risk lesions. Metastasis from an SCC of this size is relatively uncommon, but depends on the grade of tumour and depth of infiltration. Those greater than 4mm in depth are especially prone to metastasize. Combined photodynamic therapy with CO_2 laser has been shown to be effective in selected cases of BCC. PDT monotherapy is also effective in small and superficial lesions, and is also especially useful in cases of Bowen's disease. However, PDT is not indicated at present in the management of SCC. Experimental evidence does, however, show some potential for non-surgical modalities in the treatment of melanoma and SCC.

References

1. Motley R, Kersey P, Lawrence C; British Association of Dermatologists; British Association of Plastic Surgeons. Multiprofessional guidelines for the management of

the patient with primary cutaneous squamous cell carcinoma. *Br J Plast Surg* 2003; 56(2): 85-91. (Dermatologists use this reference: *Br J Dermatol* 2002; 146(1): 18-25. which is the same article).

36 D.

It leads to a definite increase in overall survival. D is false. Sentinel node biopsy remains a controversial topic. It has not reached the status of a universal gold standard, and current evidence has not yet proven an increased overall survival to date. It is a powerful prognostic indicator and allows improved staging, and is incorporated into the 2002 AJCC melanoma staging. Readers are recommended to keep up-to-date with progress with regard to this topic. The evidence and research may soon change in the near future and this is a hot topic for debate in examinations.

References

1.   Stone C, Ed. *The evidence for plastic surgery*. Shrewsbury, UK: tfm publishing Ltd, 2008.

37 B.

A better prognosis exists for a stage IIIA melanoma than for a IIC melanoma at 5 years. A better prognosis exists for a stage IIIA melanoma than for a IIC melanoma. The AJCC classification 2001 [1] gives 5-year survival for IIC tumours as 45% and IIIA as 69%. Based on 2008 AJCC data, the figures are 53% and 78%, respectively [2]. The 2009 AJCC guidelines are due for publication shortly. This highlights the prognostic significance of tumour thickness and ulceration.

References

1.   Balch CM, Buzaid AC, Soong SJ, Atkins MB, Cascinelli N, Coit DG, Fleming ID, Gershenwald JE, Houghton A Jr, Kirkwood JM, McMasters KM, Mihm MF, Morton DL, Reintgen DS, Ross MI, Sober A, Thompson JA, Thompson JF. Final version of the American Joint Committee on Cancer Staging system for cutaneous melanoma. *J Clin Oncol* 2001; 19(16): 3635-48.

2.   Balch CM, *et al*. In: *Cutaneous melanoma*, 5th ed. Balch, Houghton, Sober, Soong, Atkins & Thompson, Eds. St. Louis, USA: Quality Medical Publishing Inc, 2008; Chapter 4: 75.

38 A.

A patient with a 0.7mm lesion has at least a 10% risk of death by 10 years. The 10-year survival for a T1a (stage 1A) melanoma is 88%, the 5-year survival being 95%.

References

1.   Balch CM, Buzaid AC, Soong SJ, Atkins MB, Cascinelli N, Coit DG, Fleming ID, Gershenwald JE, Houghton A Jr, Kirkwood JM, McMasters KM, Mihm MF, Morton DL, Reintgen DS, Ross MI, Sober A, Thompson JA, Thompson JF. Final version of the American Joint Committee on Cancer Staging system for cutaneous melanoma. *J Clin Oncol* 2001; 19(16): 3635-48.

39 D.

Is more common in brunettes than blondes. In relation to risk by hair colour, the relative risk compared to black hair is: redhead - 3.6 times higher, brunette - 2.8 times higher, blonde - 2.4 times higher. The risk of transformation of a giant hairy naevus is variably quoted as between 1 and 40%. However, it is now thought to be well below a 10% lifetime risk. Delay in diagnosis can lead to a worse prognosis in those with black skin. Spitz naevi occur in children and young adults. The unfortunate and now obsolete synonym, juvenile melanoma, was applied to the seminal works on these tumours. They are not malignant lesions and should be differentiated from the rare cases of true melanoma in this age group. There is some grey in this area, and there are reports of an entity termed 'malignant Spitz naevus'.

References

1.   Gnepp DR. *Diagnostic surgical pathology of the head and neck*, 2nd ed. Saunders-Elsevier, 2009: 1050-1.
2.   Spitz S. Melanomas of childhood. *Am J Pathol* 1948; 24: 591-609.
3.   Smith KJ, *et al*. Spindle cell and epithelioid cell nevi with atypia and metastasis (malignant Spitz nevus). *Am J Surg Pathol* 1980; 13: 931-9.

40 D.

It has an 88% 10-year survival if <1mm Breslow thickness. Superficial spreading melanoma is the commonest subtype. *In situ* melanoma has a 100% survival. It is most commonly found on the trunk and head of men and the lower extremity of women. In general it is commoner in men.

References

1. Balch CM, Buzaid AC, Soong SJ, Atkins MB, Cascinelli N, Coit DG, Fleming ID, Gershenwald JE, Houghton A Jr, Kirkwood JM, McMasters KM, Mihm MF, Morton DL, Reintgen DS, Ross MI, Sober A, Thompson JA, Thompson JF. Final version of the American Joint Committee on Cancer Staging system for cutaneous melanoma. *J Clin Oncol* 2001; 19(16): 3635-48.

41 B.

Can be treated successfully with photodynamic therapy. Photodynamic therapy consists of treatment with a photosensitizer such as 5-aminolevulinic acid, and the application of narrow wavelength light or a laser for activation and cellular destruction. It can be painful during photoactivation. It can be used on a range of malignant and premalignant skin conditions, especially actinic keratosis, Bowen's disease (squamous carcinoma *in situ*) and BCC. The modality does not provide histopathological confirmation of clearance, but can yield cure rates in superficial lesions approaching those of surgical excision with excellent cosmesis. The commonest complication is hypopigmentation.

42 C.

A 4mm margin on the face gives a cure rate of greater than 90%. Metastasis is extremely rare, but reported. The commonest lower lip tumour is squamous carcinoma. Pigmented BCCs are a well-recognised subtype. BCCs are familial in Gorlin's syndrome as an autosomal dominant trait, although up to a third are *de novo* mutations.

Section 8 questions

Paediatric plastic surgery

1   In obstetrical brachial plexus paralysis (OBPP):

A.   Primary suture without tension is frequently possible.
B.   Internal neurotization should be attempted only when C5 and C6 are ruptured.
C.   Motion of the extremity should be started immediately after surgery to avoid stiffness.
D.   Babies who do not recover biceps function by the age of 3 months should be considered for immediate operation.
E.   Physiotherapy can be discontinued once the biceps start to flex the elbow.

2   Which statement concerning haemangioma is incorrect?

A.   Present in 10% of newborns with white skin.
B.   Occurs in female infants three times more commonly than in male infants.
C.   Incidence is higher in premature infants.
D.   Is rarely hereditary.
E.   Precursor (herald) marks are present in approximately 50% of children who develop a haemangioma.

3 The common starting dosage for the treatment of infantile haemangioma with oral prednisolone:

A. 0.002-0.004mg/kg/day.
B. 0.02-0.04mg/kg/day.
C. 0.2-0.4mg/kg/day.
D. 2-4mg/kg/day.
E. 20-40mg/kg/day.

4 Which is not a feature of Klippel-Trenaunay syndrome (KTS)?

A. Limb overgrowth.
B. Venous varicosities.
C. Limb undergrowth.
D. Cerebriform palmar hyperplasia.
E. Lymphatic malformation.

5 A 7-year-old boy has hypernasality and velopharyngeal incompetence. He underwent repair of a ventricular septal defect at birth and repair of a cleft palate at age 9 months. His mother says that he has had difficulties with language learning. Physical examination shows upward slanting of the palpebral fissures, a broad nasal root, a small mouth, and a thin upper lip. Which of the following studies is most likely to lead to a diagnosis in this patient?

A. Measurement of serum creatine kinase level.
B. Chromosomal karyotyping.
C. Fluorescent in situ hybridisation (FISH) analysis.
D. MR angiography.
E. None of these.

6 The following is true about otoplasty:

A. Glue can be used effectively instead of head bandages.
B. Conchal reduction should be undertaken using an anterior approach in most cases.
C. Closed techniques of cartilage scoring have high recurrence rates.
D. Splinting of the ear after birth to correct prominent ears is an old wives' tale and simply does not work.
E. Suture techniques have lower complication rates than cartilage scoring techniques.

7 A frontonasal encephalocele commonly causes:

A. Hypertelorism.
B. Double vision.
C. Telecanthus.
D. Frontal sinus enlargement.
E. Nasal shortening.

8 Which is false regarding Treacher-Collins syndrome?

A. It is the same as Franceschetti syndrome and mandibulofacial dysostosis.
B. It is relatively rare with an incidence of 1:25,000-1:50,000.
C. It is equivalent to combined Tessier clefts 7, 8 and 9.
D. Cleft palate is often a feature.
E. Angle class II malocclusion is a feature.

9 A 7-year-old has cryptotia. Which of the following operative techniques is most appropriate for correction?

A. Advancement of the third crus of the antihelix.
B. Partial detachment of the folded segment of helical cartilage from the scapha and repositioning of the helix with sutures.

C.   Placement of sutures from the conchal bowl to the mastoid fascia.
D.   Rasping of the anterior surface of the antihelical cartilage to create the antihelix.
E.   Separation of the superior auricle from the temporal skin with placement of a retro-auricular skin graft.

10 A neonate has C5-6 brachial plexus palsy at birth. Complete recovery of function is most likely in this patient if some activity is demonstrated in the deltoid and biceps muscles by how many months of age?

A.   3 months.
B.   5 months.
C.   6 months.
D.   8 months.
E.   12 months.

11 Regarding hemifacial atrophy, which is correct?

A.   Is due to a chromosome abnormality (11p3).
B.   Is due to a chromosome abnormality (15q11).
C.   Is best monitored using thermography.
D.   Should be treated surgically within 6 months of diagnosis.
E.   Osteotomies are not indicated as this is only a soft-tissue disease.

12 With regards to hypospadias surgery:

A.   Flip-flap (Mathieu) repair is a two-stage repair.
B.   Meatal advancement with glanuloplasty incorporated (MAGPI) and Snodgrass (tubularised incised plate [TIP]) repairs are BOTH single-stage repairs.
C.   Full thickness skin grafts must come from the buccal mucosa.
D.   Homan's test is critical before commencing surgery.
E.   Circumcision should be undertaken as part of the first stage of Bracka's repair.

13 During assessment of velopharyngeal incompetence, the following patterns of velopharyngeal closure can be seen on videofluoroscopy:

A. Coronal.
B. Sagittal.
C. Sphincteric.
D. Sphinteric with Passavant's ridge.
E. None of the above.

14 A harlequin orbit is diagnostic of:

A. Sagittal craniosynostosis.
B. Coronal craniosynostosis.
C. Fibrous dysplasia.
D. Metopic craniosynostosis.
E. Cranial neurofibromatosis.

15 Clefts:

A. Are more common in black races than Asians.
B. Are more common in white races than Asians.
C. Are more common in white races than black races.
D. Are less common in younger siblings of those with cleft lip and palate.
E. None of the above.

16 Which strategy is least favourable for dealing with velopharyngeal incompetence?

A. Hynes pharyngoplasty.
B. Intravelar veloplasty.
C. Furlow palatoplasty.
D. Orticochea pharyngoplasty.
E. Posterior pharyngeal wall augmentation.

17 The overall incidence of bifid uvula in the population is:

A.   Between 1:100 and 1:70.
B.   Between 1:12000 and 1:1000.
C.   Between 1:12000 and 1:10000.
D.   Between 1:35 and 1:25.
E.   None of the above.

18 Which French surgeon was the first to use the buried skin strip to repair hypospadias?

A.   Byars.
B.   Duplay.
C.   Anger.
D.   Cecil.
E.   Novè-Josserand.

19 Which method used to repair hypospadias is the odd one out?

A.   Ombredanne.
B.   Byars.
C.   Cecil-Culp.
D.   Horton-Devine.
E.   Duplay.

20 Who was the first to advocate including the palatal periosteum in flaps used to repair cleft palate?

A.   von Langenbeck.
B.   Hulke.
C.   Dieffenbach.
D.   Billroth.
E.   Fergusson.

21 Microtia is associated with all except:

A.   Deformity of the middle ear.
B.   Deformity of the cochlea.
C.   Psychological distress.
D.   Mandibular hypoplasia.
E.   Treacher-Collins syndrome.

22 Cleft lip:

A.   With or without cleft palate is different in aetiology to isolated cleft palate.
B.   Is associated with a 75% risk of further congenital abnormalities.
C.   Is inherited as an X-linked trait.
D.   Is best treated after the age of 3 years.
E.   When extending posterior to the incisive foramen is sometimes referred to as a complex cleft lip.

23 Pfeiffer syndrome consists of all except:

A.   Tower skull.
B.   Midface hypoplasia.
C.   Brachydactyly.
D.   Cleft palate.
E.   Hypertelorism.

24 Strategies for preventing complications in suture-based otoplasty include all except:

A.   Use of a round-bodied needle.
B.   Use of a postauricular fascial flap.
C.   Use of a polyglycolic suture material.
D.   Careful haemostasis.
E.   Use of specific forceps to handle cartilage.

25 In cleft surgery, the following is true:

A. Two methods of bilateral cleft lip repair include the Manchester repair and the Millard repair.
B. Two popular methods of unilateral cleft lip repair include the Manchester repair and the Millard repair.
C. Tajima, McComb and Matsuma are all names related to surgery of the lip itself.
D. Simonart's band affects the lateral aspect of the lower lip.
E. Simonart's band affects the medial aspect of the lower lip.

26 The optic nerve is most endangered in the following:

A. Neurofibromatosis.
B. Coronal craniosynostosis.
C. Fibrous dysplasia.
D. Thyrotoxicosis.
E. Hemifacial microsomia.

27 Isolated cleft palate:

A. Is a congenital defect of the primary palate posterior to the incisive foramen.
B. Is a congenital defect of the hard palate anterior to the incisive foramen.
C. Can occur as submucous clefts which often present only with speech abnormalities.
D. Is twice as common in males.
E. Is syndromic in less than 10% of cases.

28 The facial bipartition technique is best suited to the correction of:

A.   Crouzon's deformity.
B.   Hemifacial microsomia.
C.   Frontonasal encephalocele.
D.   Apert's syndrome.
E.   Mandibular prognathism.

29 The incidence of hydrocephalus in craniofacial dysostosis patients is:

A.   10%.
B.   20%.
C.   30%.
D.   50%.
E.   70%.

30 The LeFort II osteotomy is limited in value but may be indicated in:

A.   Thyrotoxic exorbitism.
B.   Binder's syndrome.
C.   Apert's syndrome.
D.   Crouzon's syndrome.
E.   Hypertelorism.

31 Telecanthus is defined as:

A.   Lateral displacement of the orbits.
B.   Lateral nasal displacement.
C.   Increased width of the nasal bridge line.
D.   Prominence of the supra-orbital rims.
E.   Bilateral airway blockage.

32 In relation to presurgical orthopaedics in the context of cleft lip and palate:

A. Its use is universal in severe deformities.
B. Passive devices such as the Latham appliance are commonly used.
C. Can be undertaken simply by use of an obturator.
D. Are of particular benefit by improving subsequent growth of bony and soft tissue structures but can make subsequent cleft repair more difficult.
E. Dynamic devices are often fixed to the mandible.

33 Brachycephaly is the term for:

A. A narrow skull.
B. An asymmetrical skull.
C. A long skull - anteroposterior.
D. A wide skull.
E. A skull defect.

34 Unilateral coronal craniosynostosis results in:

A. Brachycephaly.
B. Turricephaly.
C. Plagiocephaly.
D. Tower skull.
E. Scaphocephaly.

35 Premature closure of the metopic suture results in:

A. Plagiocephaly.
B. Trigonocephaly.
C. Turricephaly.
D. Brachycephaly.
E. Epilepsy attacks.

36 Hemifacial microsomia (craniofacial microsomia):

A.   Is relatively common with an incidence of 1:3000-1:5000.
B.   The mandibular hypoplasia was classified by Meurman.
C.   The OMENS classification includes a description of the spinal deformity.
D.   Osseodistraction is a last resort due to the fragility of the skeleton in these patients.
E.   Orbital dystopia is almost never seen in this group.

37 Treacher-Collins syndrome consists of all except:

A.   Lower eyelid colobomas.
B.   Malar hypoplasia.
C.   Antimongoloid palpebral fissures.
D.   Cleft palate.
E.   Micrognathia.

38 With regard to giant congenital naevi:

A.   These are defined as >20cm squared surface area.
B.   They are defined as greater than 5% body surface area.
C.   Treatments such as dermabrasion and CO_2 laser are more effective after the age of 3.
D.   The risk of malignancy is at least 50% (lifetime).
E.   None of the above is true.

39 Neonatal splintage can be used to correct (choose two):

A.   Microtia.
B.   Prominent ears.
C.   Stahl's bar.
D.   Pre-auricular tags.
E.   Darwin's tubercle.

40 Extravasation injuries with non-isotonic agents are not infrequent in infants. Which is not true regarding management of these injuries?

A.   Always remove the cannula.
B.   Hyaluronidase injection may be of benefit.
C.   Excision and grafting of the injured area may be appropriate.
D.   Stab incisions and saline flush of the area can help.
E.   The infusion pump should always be stopped.

41 Which of the following statements regarding birthmarks is true?

A.   Haemangiomas are usually present at birth.
B.   The Q-switched laser is the treatment of choice for port wine stains.
C.   35% of port wine stains involving the ophthalmic and maxillary dermatomes of the trigeminal nerve are associated with Sturge-Weber syndrome.
D.   Cystic hygroma is a form of microcyctic lymphatic malformation.
E.   "Not all haemangiomas look like strawberries, and not all strawberries are haemangiomas."

42 The superficial penile arteries that supply the skin and prepuce of the penis come directly from which artery?

A.   Superficial circumflex iliac artery.
B.   Dorsal artery of the penis.
C.   Internal pudendal artery.
D.   External pudendal artery.
E.   Obturator artery.

43 Retrognathia is the term used for:

A.   Nasal enlargement.
B.   Mandibular enlargement.
C.   Mandibular protrusion.
D.   Maxillary retrusion.
E.   Mandibular retrusion.

44 Trimming the margins and performing a straight line closure of the cleft lip was routine until this surgeon introduced his lateral triangular flap method. Who was he?

A.   Veau.
B.   Velpeau.
C.   Mirault.
D.   Simonartz.
E.   Dieffenbach.

45 All are true regarding submucous cleft palate except:

A.   Diagnostic signs include a bifid uvula.
B.   Diagnostic signs include notching of the hard palate.
C.   Diagnostic signs include muscular diastasis of the soft palate with intact mucosa.
D.   The pterygoid hamulus is absent.
E.   Levator veli palatini insertion is displaced.

46 In obstetrical brachial plexus palsy (OBPP):

A. 50% of babies proceed to full spontaneous recovery within 3 months.
B. Some elbow flexion is present.
C. The branches of the posterior cord are unaffected.
D. The Oberlin's transfer can be a useful procedure.
E. Horner's sign is usually present.

47 A simple 'ridge' of mucosa created on the back of the pharynx of cleft patients to try and reduce nasal escape is sometimes called after a surgeon. Who was he?

A. Pigott.
B. Passavant.
C. Hynes
D. Rosselli.
E. Orticochea.

48 Classifications, scoring systems and syndromes that are relevant to cleft lip and palate and its management include all except:

A. GOSPAS scale.
B. Kernahan's classification.
C. LAHSHAL classification.
D. Kubitza's scale.
E. Catch-22 syndrome.

49 Which is true regarding pilomatrixoma (calcifying epithelioma of Malherbe)?

A. They are occasionally malignant.

B. They are commonest on the back.
C. They are usually at least 3cm in size.
D. There is actually no calcification on histology.
E. They are fixed to overlying skin.

50 'Straight-line' techniques for the repair of cleft lip include those described by:

A. Both Rose-Thompson and Millard.
B. Both Millard and Le Mesurier.
C. Both Wynn and Tennison-Randall.
D. None except one of the above named.
E. None of the above.

51 The following is true about the Salter-Harris classification of paediatric fractures:

A. Type I has a good prognosis.
B. Type II includes a fracture line through the epiphysis.
C. Type III includes a fracture line through the metaphysis.
D. Type IV is a crush injury.
E. None are true.

52 The following are associated with hypospadias except:

A. Scrotal bipartition.
B. Chordee.
C. Both inguinal hernia and undescended testes.
D. Androgen hypersensitivity.
E. Environmental oestrogens.

53 The following is true regarding cleft palate surgery:

A.   The Veau-Kilner-Wardill technique is also described as the 'push forward' technique.
B.   The von Langenbeck technique involves raising a unipedicled flap.
C.   Intravelar veloplasty involves repair of the nasal mucosa.
D.   The Furlow technique is a V-Y plasty.
E.   The Furlow technique is a W-plasty.

54 Prominent ear correction:

A.   Should ensure the antihelix marginally projects more than the helix.
B.   Can often be corrected with splitage at 2-3 years of age.
C.   Is best undertaken at age 5.
D.   Using the Mustardé and Chongchet (anterior scoring) techniques were both described in 1963 in the *British Journal of Plastic Surgery*.
E.   Should never be undertaken unless definite psychological trauma can be demonstrated in a child.

Section 8 answers

Paediatric plastic surgery

1 D.

Babies who do not recover biceps function by the age of 3 months should be considered for immediate operation.

Also note:

- Primary suture without tension is rarely possible. Nerve grafting is usually necessary for root or trunk ruptures.
- In the presence of root avulsions an internal neurotization should be attempted between different roots, particularly as children seem to have a far greater capacity to accommodate to differential neurotizations.
- When it is not possible to perform an internal neurotization, an external neurotization can be performed using one or more of the following donor nerves in the following order of preference: the pectoral nerves, the intercostal nerves and the accessory nerve.
- The reconstruction should be protected from excessive motion for the first 3 weeks.
- Physiotherapy should be continued up to 2 years of age but then continued by the parents in the form of play and activities of daily living.
- Secondary surgery can be considered when it is clear that recovery following reconstruction is no longer progressing.

References

1. Gilbert A. Primary repair of the obstetrical plexus. *Indian Journal of Plastic Surgery* 2005; 38(1): 34-42.

2   A.

Present in 10% of newborns with white skin. This statement is incorrect; haemangiomas are present in approximately 10% of white skinned children by the age of 1 year, but only 1-2% of newborns. Female infants are three times more likely to have haemangiomas, and the incidence is increased in premature neonates. They occur in all races but less commonly in African or Asian skin. Although traditionally considered to be sporadic, autosomal dominant segregation within families has been described but rare. Haemangiomas present with a variety of precursor lesions in approximately 50% of cases and these can be present at birth.

3   D.

2-4mg/kg/day. Corticosteroids are the mainstay of therapy for haemangiomas that require treatment, most commonly administered orally, but intra-lesional and topical preparations can be useful. They are most useful in the proliferative phase. 2-4mg/kg/day is the standard starting regime but some advocate up to 5mg/kg/day and the therapy is usually continued for several months and gradually tapered as tolerated.

4   D.

Cerebriform palmar hyperplasia. This is not a feature of Klippel-Trenaunay syndrome (KTS). KTS is a sporadic disorder characterised by a triad of vascular malformation, venous varicosity and growth disturbance of soft tissue or bone. Capillary malformation of the port wine type is the most common vascular malformation but can be present with underlying lymphatic malformation. Overgrowth (hyperplasia) is most common but undergrowth can also occur in the affected limb. Cerebriform palmar hyperplasia is a feature of Proteus syndrome, another overgrowth syndrome.

5   C.

Fluorescent in situ hybridisation (FISH) analysis. This is the classic test to diagnose velocardiofacial syndrome, otherwise known as Di George syndrome, Shprintzen's syndrome and catch 22 syndrome (chromosome locus 22q11.2; C - cardia, A - abnormal facies, T - thymic aplasia, C - cleft palate, H - hypocalcaemia). Inheritence is usually sporadic.

References

1.   Shprintzen RJ. Velocardiofacial syndrome. *Otolaryngeal Chin North Am* 2000; 33: 1217-40.

2.   Raymond GV. Craniofacial genetics and dysmorphology. In: *Plastic surgery: indications, operations, and outcomes.* Achauer BM, Eriksson E, Guyuron B, Coleman JJ, Russell RC, Vander Kolk CA, Eds. St. Louis, USA: Mosby, 2000.

6   A.

Glue can be used effectively instead of head bandages. Glue for postoperative splinting in the context of suture techniques of prominent ear correction was first described in 2008 and can be used instead of head bandages. This removes the need for an office appointment for removal of head bandages, patients can shower after the first postoperative day, and girls in particular can wear their hair long hiding any stigmata of surgery immediately postoperatively. A finer subcuticular skin closure can also be used, and bandages falling off are no longer an issue. An 'internal corset' using an anteriorly-based fascial flap can provide further support to the ear in this context [1, 2]. Conchal reduction is best undertaken from a posterior approach to hide the scar, although anterior approaches have been described for this purpose and also for harvest of cartilage grafts without undue cosmetic morbidity. Closed scoring techniques such as popularised by Stenstrom are not particularly associated with any increased risk of complications. Many consider suture techniques to have lower complication rates than cartilage scoring techniques in otoplasty. There is no incontrovertible evidence for this and a number of groups have published excellent results with low complications [3]. When severe complications occur, they anecdotally seem to be more prevalent in open cartilage scoring techniques, although this is a controversial and unproven statement. Splinting of the ear within weeks of birth can be effective for correction of prominent ears due to some residual plasticity of the ear cartilage. Skin glue can also be used for this task [4] as well as a number of proprietary or custom-made appliances.

References

1. Shokrollahi K, Cooper MA, Hiew LY. A new strategy for otoplasty. *J Plast Reconstr Surg* 2009; 62: 774-81.

2. Shokrollahi K, Tanner B. 'Glue ear': beginning of the end for head bandages after prominent ear correction? *J Plast Reconstr Aesthet Surg* 2008; 61(9): 1077.

3. Caouette-Laberge L, Guay N, Bortoluzzi P, Belleville CB. Otoplasty: anterior scoring technique and results in 500 cases. *Plast Reconstr Surg* 2000; 105(2): 504-15.

4. Scrimshaw G. The 30-second otoplasty. *Ann Plast Surg* 1983; 10(1): 86-7.

7   C.

Telecanthus.

8   C.

It is equivalent to combined Tessier clefts 7, 8 and 9. C is false. It is actually equivalent to a 6, 7 and 8 cleft. This is an autosomal dominant condition with an abnormality of chromosme 5 first described by Treacher Collins in 1900. Colobomas of the lower eyelid are common, as is cleft palate. Ear abnormalities (microtia) are seen and there is an overbite malocclusion.

9   E.

Separation of the superior auricle from the temporal skin with placement of a retro-auricular skin graft.

References

1. Furnas D. The correction of prominent ears by concha-mastoid sutures. *Plast Reconstr Surg* 1968; 42(3): 189-94.

2.   Leber D. Ear reconstruction. In: *Textbook of plastic, maxillofacial and reconstruction surgery*, 2nd ed. Georgiade GS, Georgiade N, Riefkohl R, Levin LS, Eds. Baltimore, USA: Williams & Wilkins, 1992: 497.
3.   Mustardé J. The correction of prominent ears using mattress sutures. *Br J Plast Surg* 1963; 16: 170.
4.   Sugino H. Surgical correction of Stahl's ear using the cartilage turnover and rotating method. *Plast Reconstr Surg* 1989; 83(1): 160-4.
5.   Tanzer R. The constricted (cup and lop) ear. *Plast Reconstr Surg* 1975; 55(4): 406-15.

10 A.

3 months.

References

1.   Clarke HM, Cuttis CG. An approach to obstetrical brachial plexus oinjuries. *Hand Clin* 1995; 11: 563-81.
2.   Gilbert A. Long-term evaluation of brachial plexus surgery in obstetrical palsy. *Hand Clin* 1995; 11: 583-55.
3.   Michelow BJ, Clarke HM, Curtis CG, Zuker RM, Seifu Y, Andrews D, Laurent J. The natural history of obstetrical brachial plexus palsy. *Plast Reconstr Surg* 1994; 93(4): 675-81.

11 C.

Is best monitored using thermography. Thermography is the best modality to monitor the activity of the disease. Hemifacial atrophy is also referred to as Romberg's disease or Parry-Romberg disease. It is unilateral and sporadic with an onset usually between early childhood and late teens/early twenties. A classic 'coup de sabre' deformity is occasionally seen, and other atrophic changes involve the eye, hair, skin, soft tissue and bone. Treatment options include fat transfer, free or pedicled flaps including fascial flaps - classically parascapular, scapular, omental and ALT. Surgery should be delayed until the disease is no longer active.

12 B.

Meatal advancement with glanuloplasty incorporated (MAGPI) and Snodgrass (tubularised incised plate [TIP]) repairs are BOTH single-stage repairs.

13 E.

None of the above. These patterns of velopharyngeal closure are seen when assessed by nasendoscopy. This procedure is undertaken with the patient awake to enable co-operation and assessment. In general, coronal patterns of velopharyngeal closure are best treated with sphincter pharyngoplasty whereas sagittal patterns are best treated with posterior pharyngeal flaps.

14 B.

Coronal craniosynostosis. This is due to dysplasia of the sphenoid bone deforming the middle cranial fossa and causing proptosis.

15 C.

Are more common in white races than black races.

16 E.

Posterior pharyngeal wall augmentation. This is the least favourable strategy. Hynes from Sheffield UK delivered his Hunterian Oration on his sphincter pharyngoplasty technique in 1953. This involved use of the salpingopharyngeus muscle, but it was developed to later include a greater amount of musculature including palatopharyngeus. Orticochea from Bogota in Colombia, described an inferiorly-based pharyngeal flap in conjunction with sphincter pharyngoplasty. Intravelar veloplasty has been popularised by Sommerlad. These, along with Furlow's double-opposing Z-plasty soft palate repair, are useful strategies for velopharyngeal incompetence. Veau's push-back repair lengthens the soft palate and has theoretical advantages, but has fallen out of favour as it causes unacceptable midfacial hypoplasia. Augmentation of the posterior pharyngeal wall with fillers ranging from Teflon® to autologous fat have not, as yet, been successful to the extent that they have been widely adopted.

17 A.

Between 1:100 and 1:70.

18 B.

Duplay. The Frenchman, Simon Duplay, was the first to use a buried skin strip in 1874. Instead of sewing it into a tunnel he allowed it to tube itself to form the new urethra and covered it with lateral flaps. The method was popularised in England by Denis Browne at Great Ormond Street Hospital.

19 D.

Horton-Devine. Horton and Devine devised a single-stage correction; all the others are two-stage or multi-stage.

20 A.

von Langenbeck. Dieffenbach was the first to repair the defect in the bone of the hard palate in 1826 by performing an osteotomy on the palatal bones and shifting a composite flap of bone and mucosa medially but von Langenbeck saw the potential of including just periosteum with mucosal flaps and designed a special elevator to achieve this end. He presented his modification of Dieffenbach's method in 1861 in Berlin.

21 B.

Deformity of the cochlea. This is not associated with microtia. Microtia is hypoplasia of the external ear with an incidence of approximately 1:5000, more commonly occurring on the right. The inner ear is rarely involved, but conduction deafness is often found. Treatment can be with a prosthesis which can be glued on or osseointegrated (Branemark®), or through ear reconstruction.

22 A.

With or without cleft palate is different in aetiology to isolated cleft palate.

23 D.

Cleft palate. This is not present in Pfeiffer syndrome.

24 C.

Use of a polyglycolic suture material. This is incorrect; polyglycolic sutures are dissolvable and a permanent suture should be used for pinnaplasty. Common choices include Ethibond® and clear Prolene®. A round-bodied needle prevents possible chondral microfractures from cutting needles along which sutures can pull through. A postauricular fascial flap can be based posteriorly [1] or anteriorly [2]. Brown forceps prevent damage to cartilage during manipulation.

References

1. Horlock N, Misra A, Gault DT. The postauricular fascial flap as an adjunct to Mustardé and Furnas type otoplasty. *Plast Reconstr Surg* 2001; 108(6): 1487-90; discussion 1491

2. Shokrollahi K, Cooper MA, Hiew LY. A new strategy for otoplasty. *J Plast Reconstr Surg* 2009; 62: 774-81.

25 A.

Two methods of bilateral cleft lip repair include the Manchester repair and the Millard repair. Tajima, McComb and Matsuma are nasal repairs. Simonart's band affects the upper lip.

26 C.

Fibrous dysplasia. Craniofacial fibrous dysplasia ranges from mild to severe disease and is divided into 4 zones. Zone 1 is orbital, zone 2 is hair-bearing cranium, zone 3 is the cranial base and zone 4 is the maxilla and mandible. There is a small risk of malignant transformation. Orbital disease can cause proptosis, optic nerve atrophy and blindness.

27 C.

Can occur as submucous clefts which often present only with speech abnormalities.

28 D.

Apert's syndrome. The main cranial feature of this syndrome is bicoronal synostosis. The aims of treatment include addressing form and function. Crisis management involves treatment of ocular exposure including tarsorrhaphy or early fronto-orbital advancement, treatment of raised intracranial pressure with ventriculoperitoneal (VP) shunts, and treatment of airway compromise. Midface hypoplasia can be treated by distraction or Le Fort 3 osteotomy/advancement or Monasterio's technique of Monobloc advancement. The treatment of the cranium is often cranial vault remodelling and fronto-orbital advancement but facial bipartition has a number of advantages in selected cases.

29 A.

10%.

30 B.

Binder's syndrome. Binder's syndrome is a sporadic congenital malformation with nasomaxillary hypoplasia. Le Fort II or III osteotomies may be indicated depending on presentation with simultaneous bone grafting. Rhinoplasty is usually undertaken at a later stage.

31 C.

Increased width of the nasal bridge line. Increased width of the nasal bridge line is due to the increased distance from the medial canthus to the nose.

32 C.

Can be undertaken simply by use of an obturator. Presurgical orthopaedics is controversial and not universally accepted.

33 D.

A wide skull. It is most commonly caused by bicoronal synostosis as in Crouzon's syndrome or Apert's. The skull is often tower-shaped and high and often referred to as turribrachycephaly.

34 C.

Plagiocephaly. Plagiocephaly literally means 'twisted skull'. This can be frontal plagiocephaly from unilateral coronal synostosis or occipital due to unilateral lambdoidal synostosis.

35 B.

Trigonocephaly.

36 A.

Is relatively common with an incidence of 1:3000-1:5000. The mandibular hypoplasia was classified by Pruzansky (Muerman described ear deformity). OMENS is another classification which describes ocular, mandibular, ear, nerve and soft tissue deficiencies. Osseodistraction is first-line treatment for most skeletal correction. Orbital dystopia is common.

37 E.

Micrognathia.

38 B.

They are defined as greater than 5% body surface area. Giant congenital naevi are defined as >5% surface area or 20cm in *diameter.* Because the naevi are more superficial and mature (travel deeper) with time, early treatment with ablative modalities may be more efficacious. The malignant potential is controversial with widely quoted rates from 2-40% (approximate) but significant evidence points towards a lesser risk than previously thought and 50% would be an exaggerated risk.

39 B and C.

Prominent ears and *Stahl's bar.*

40 A.

Always remove the cannula. This is incorrect; the cannula may be of benefit in treatment if it is kept *in situ* to help with lavage or administration of an antidote. The infusion pump should be stopped immediately if that is the source. Injection of hyaluronidase and flushes with saline through multiple stab incisions around the area can help reduce the extent of tissue damage. Excision and grafting or other methods of reconstruction may be required, but usually as a delayed procedure.

41 E.

"Not all haemangiomas look like strawberries, and not all strawberries are haemangiomas." Anon.

42 D.

External pudendal artery. External pudendal arteries (can be superior and inferior) arise from the femoral artery and anastomose to form the superficial arterial system supplying the prepuce and skin. The internal pudendal, a branch of the internal iliac, supplies the dorsal artery of the penis, and the deep artery of the penis which in turn supplies the corpus cavernosum.

43 E.

Mandibular retrusion.

44 C.

Mirault. In 1844, Germanicus Mirault (1796-1879) used a triangular flap from the lateral side and introduced it into a horizontal incision on the medial margin of the cleft to break up the vertical scar. His contribution was recognised by Victor Veau a century later: "Mirault was the genius of cleft lip surgery."

45 D.

The pterygoid hamulus is absent. This is incorrect; the pterygoid hamulus is NOT absent.

46 D.

The Oberlin's transfer can be a useful procedure. Narakas has classified obstetric brachial palsy into the following four groups:

- Group 1 represents classic Erb (C5/C6) palsy with initial absence of shoulder abduction, shoulder rotation, elbow flexion and forearm supination.
- Group 2 includes C7 with absence of wrist and finger extension.
- Group 3 is a flail extremity without a Horner's syndrome.
- Group 4 is the most severe group - a flail extremity with a Horner's syndrome. This indicates a very poor prognosis. Presence of a Horner's syndrome indicates a preganglionic injury to the lower plexus.

Classical Erb's palsy involves only C5/C6 (c.50%) but it is also common to have C5/C6/C7 involvement. A recent study has shown that 91% of palsies fall into these categories. In group 1, approximately 90% proceed to full recovery, with some evidence of recovery by 3 months. Biceps and brachialis are innervated by C5/C6 and so elbow flexion is absent. Branches of the posterior cord are affected, particularly the branches of the axillary nerve (C5/C6). The Oberlin's transfer involves moving a fascicle from the ulnar nerve to the motor branch to biceps and can be useful in C5/C6 avulsion.

47 B.

Passavant. Gustav Passavant (1813-1893) attempted to reduce nasal escape by making a ridge of mucosa from a quadrilateral flap on the back wall of the palate in 1878 but its effects were short lived. Passavant's ridge can be a naturally occurring phenomenon due to constriction of the levator veli palatini and superior constrictors.

48 D.

Kubitza's scale. This is incorrect. GOSPAS is the Great Ormond Street Hospital Speech Assessment tool. Kernahan and Stark described the striped Y classification for cleft lip and palate assessment. Catch-22 syndrome is synonymous with Di George syndrome, velocardofacial syndrome and Shprintzen's syndrome and is due to a deletion at the 22q11.2 chromosome locus. The LAHSHAL classification of clefts was described by Kriens.

49 E.

They are fixed to overlying skin. These common benign tumours are mainly seen in children and are benign. They are common on the face and are usually less than 1cm in size. There is calcification and substantial keratinisation on histology.

50 E.

None of the above.

51 A.

Type I has a good prognosis. Type I Salter-Harris fractures generally have a good prognosis and can be thought of as 'slipped' epiphyses. There are five types, Type V being a crush injury of the growth plate. Type II involves the metaphysis, Type III the epiphysis, and Type IV both the metaphysis and epiphysis.

52 D.

Androgen hypersensitivity.

53 C.

Intravelar veloplasty involves repair of the nasal mucosa. The Veau-Kilner-Wardill technique is a push-back technique, the von Langenbeck technique is a bepidicled technique and Furlow described the double-opposing Z-plasty.

54 D.

Using the Mustardé and Chongchet (anterior scoring) techniques were both described in 1963 in the British Journal of Plastic Surgery. It is best undertaken after age 5 when the ear has achieved 80% of its adult size. To avoid an 'overcorrected' look the antihelix should not be more prominent than the helix. Otoplasty is a relatively simple operation in experienced hands, and if parents and child are keen for surgery, this is entirely reasonable.

References

1.   Chongchet V. A method of antihelix reconstruction. *Br J Plast Surg* 1963; 16: 268-72.

2.   Mustardé C.The correction of prominent ears using simple mattress sutures. *Br J Plast Surg* 1963; 16: 170-8.

3.   Shokrollahi K, Kaney SJ. Psychological considerations in patient selection for pinnaplasty. *J Plast Reconstr Aesthet Surg* 2009; 62(1): 118.

Section 9 questions

History of plastic surgery

1 In which country during the 3rd century BC was the first cleft lip repair performed?

A. Egypt.
B. Greece.
C. China.
D. Roman Italy.
E. Etruscan Italy.

2 First introduced in 1958, the widely accepted classification of clefts, which uses the incisive foramen as a reference point, was described by?

A. Reidy.
B. Kernahan.
C. Veau.
D. Pöhlmann.
E. Oborne.

3 The 1561 book, *Traites des Hernies*, by Pierre Franco contains work on:

A. Clefts.
B. Amputations.
C. Parotid tumours.
D. None of these.
E. All of these.

263

4   Which London surgeon used a skin graft introduced with a specially designed trocar to repair hypospadias?

A.   Browne.
B.   McIndoe.
C.   Matthews.
D.   Mowlem.
E.   Watson.

5   The following statements concerning the history of plastic surgery are true except:

A.   Tagliacozzi was born in Bologna in 1545.
B.   Kilner was the Nuffield Professor of Plastic Surgery in Oxford.
C.   Tord Skoog was appointed Professor of Plastic Surgery in Uppsala in 1960.
D.   Sushruta is credited with being the first to perform nasal reconstruction.
E.   Sir Harold Gillies described the full thickness skin graft.

6   Who was the Frenchman in charge of the Military Hospital, Val de Grace, in Paris, France, during WWI?

A.   Morestin.
B.   Escoffier.
C.   Varenne.
D.   Soyer.
E.   Tirel.

7 Which German Jew, whose reputation is based on his rhinoplasty technique, avoided Hitler's persecution in the 1930s because of his surgical skills?

A. Israel.
B. Joseph.
C. Weisinger.
D. Jacobs.
E. Natvig.

8 In 1819, Sir Astley Cooper performed what was probably the first skin flap used to repair a defect outside the face. What did he repair with this flap?

A. A defect after skin cancer excision on the trunk.
B. A urethral fistula.
C. A defect of the neck after an ulcerating infection.
D. A wound on the lower limb.
E. None of these.

9 Which London surgeon used 'beads and stops' in his hypospadias repair?

A. McIndoe.
B. Gillies.
C. Browne.
D. Mowlem.
E. Matthews.

10 Who first described the anatomical structures which cause chordee?

A. Antyllus.
B. Lusitanus.
C. Paré.
D. Anger.
E. Galen.

11 Who wrote satirically about Tagliacozzi?

A. Molière.
B. Swift.
C. Ben Johnson.
D. Voltaire.
E. Oscar Wilde.

12 The famous 'BL' letter to a popular journal of the day concerned the patient named:

A. Carpue.
B. Colley.
C. Maharata.
D. Kooma.
E. Cowasjee.

13 Which Englishman was the first to perform a forehead flap nasal reconstruction in Europe?

A. Blanding.
B. Carpue.
C. Warren.
D. Liston.
E. Fergusson.

14 Which is the odd one out?

A. Bodenham.
B. Watson.
C. Braithwaite.
D. Padget.
E. Campbell.

15 Who said "I treated them, God healed them"?

A. Ombredanne.
B. Paré.
C. Hippocrates.
D. Galen.
E. Celsus.

16 When is Sushruta said to have written his *Samhita*?

A. 800-600 BC.
B. 100-60 BC.
C. 60 AD.
D. 300 AD.
E. 600 AD.

17 Which surgeon wrote *El Tasrif*?

A. Avicenna.
B. Albucasis.
C. Vido Vidi.
D. Oribasius
E. Apollonio.

18 Which surgeon from classical times influenced medical teaching for centuries after his death to the detriment of scientific progress?

A.   Celsus.
B.   Aquapendente.
C.   Galen.
D.   Hippocrates.
E.   Oribasius.

19 Who strongly favoured the use of cautery to control bleeding and also used it rather than the 'cold' knife?

A.   Greeks.
B.   Romans.
C.   Sicilians.
D.   Indians.
E.   Arabs.

20 Who said "Primum non nocere"?

A.   Galen.
B.   Henri de Mondeville.
C.   Guy de Chauliac.
D.   Hippocrates.
E.   Celsus.

21 Following the advances made in classical times, who kept our knowledge of medical and surgical methods alive throughout the Middle Ages?

A.   Hindus.
B.   Chinese.
C.   Arabs.

D.   French.
E.   Italians.

22 Who wrote *Humana Corporis Fabrica*?

A.   Realdus Columbus.
B.   Benedetti.
C.   da Vinci.
D.   Versalius.
E.   Mondino da Lucci.

23 In which city was Tagliacozzi the Professor of Anatomy and Surgery?

A.   Bologna.
B.   Pisa.
C.   Rome.
D.   Padua.
E.   Venice.

24 When was Tagliacozzi's book, *De Curtorum Chirurgia per Insitionem*, published?

A.   1508.
B.   1492.
C.   1597.
D.   1620.
E.   1700.

25 Prior to the publication of his seminal work on nasal reconstruction to whom did Tagliacozzi write giving details of his method?

A.   Mercurialis.
B.   Benedetti.
C.   Fallopius.
D.   Versalius.
E.   Cortesi.

26 Who wrote the classical reference text on the life story of Tagliacozzi?

A.   Carpue.
B.   Gnudi and Webster.
C.   Patterson.
D.   McDowell.
E.   Garrison.

27 Published in a 1794 *Gentleman's Magazine*, the 'BL' letter, which focused on the Indian method of rhinoplasty, drew caustic criticism from:

A.   Zeis.
B.   Dieffenbach.
C.   Delpech.
D.   von Graefe.
E.   von Langenbeck.

28 John Bell is famous for his work on:

A.   Hand function.
B.   Ligature of inaccessible arteries.
C.   Facial expression.
D.   All of these.
E.   None of these.

29 Who first described the tube pedicle?

A. Gillies.
B. McIndoe.
C. Filatov.
D. Aymard.
E. Morestin.

30 Which is the odd one out?

A. Vianeo.
B. Branca.
C. Paré.
D. von Pfolsprundt.
E. Cortesi.

31 Who wrote *On Animal Grafts* in 1804?

A. Hunter.
B. de Monceau.
C. Baronio.
D. Hooke.
E. Dutrochet.

32 Flagellation of the skin graft donor site was first reported in which country?

A. Italy.
B. Scotland.
C. India.
D. Germany.
E. Egypt.

33 Who developed the very thin skin graft?

A. Lawson.
B. Reverdin.
C. Thiersch.
D. J.M. Warren.
E. Ollier.

34 Famous victims of ear trauma include:

A. Vincent van Gogh.
B. Mike Tyson.
C. Michael Watson.
D. St Peter.
E. Saddam Hussain.

35 Who introduced 'pinch grafts'?

A. Lawson.
B. Billroth.
C. Reverdin.
D. Pollock.
E. Krause.

36 Who introduced the term 'second set phenomenon'?

A. Bert.
B. Holman.
C. Gibson.
D. Burnet.
E. Lexer.

37 Who shared the Nobel Prize for medicine in 1960?

A. Medawar.
B. Gibson.
C. Converse.
D. Kazanjian.
E. Tessier.

38 Whose graft was called a 'four-penny graft'?

A. Wadsworth.
B. Kock.
C. Lawson.
D. Krause.
E. Reverdin.

39 Apart from devising their eponymous skin grafts what do Lawson and Wolfe have in common?

A. They worked in Scotland.
B. They served in the Crimean War.
C. They were ophthalmologists.
D. They came from Eastern Europe.
E. None of these.

40 Whose work overcame the difficulties seen with full thickness grafts and very thin grafts that led to the term split skin graft?

A. Braithwaite.
B. Padget.
C. Bodenham.
D. Blair and Barret-Brown.
E. McIndoe.

41 The name of Humby is associated with:

A. Great Ormond St. Hospital.
B. Sydney Australia.
C. A graft knife.
D. All of these.
E. None of these.

42 Who is credited with inventing the skin mesher, cited as "one of those useful things invented for the wrong reason"?

A. Lanz.
B. Ponten.
C. Skoog.
D. McDowell
E. Barret-Brown.

43 Several surgeons in the 16th century were interested in cleft lip repair but who was the first to operate AND write on the subject?

A. Paré.
B. Franco.
C. de la Faye.
D. James Cook of Warwick.
E. Guillemeau.

44 What was the name of the Edinburgh medical student who described his experience of having his cleft palate repaired when 18 years old by Roux?

A. Robertson.
B. Stephenson.

C. McGregor.
D. Livington.
C. Watson.

45 The following is credited as first describing the split thickness skin graft:

A. Thiersch.
B. Wolfe.
C. Skoog.
D. Dieffenbach.
E. Branca.

46 Which surgeon conducted a very public argument with Roux about which of them was first to repair a cleft soft palate?

A. Langenbeck.
B. Vernieuil.
C. von Graefe.
D. Dieffenbach.
E. Beisemberger.

47 The following individuals are famous for their contributions to the practice of nasal reconstruction except:

A. Pfalzpaint.
B. Tagliocozzi.
C. Sushruta.
D. Branca.
E. Galen.

48 Whose name is associated with the use of small chips of bone graft sometimes used to fill cavities in bone?

A. Barth.
B. Phemister.
C. Petrov.
D. Baschkirzew.
E. Olliere.

49 Who first described the latissimus dorsi myocutaneous flap?

A. William Steward Halsted in 1882.
B. Alexis Carrel in 1912.
C. Iginio Tansini in 1896.
D. Lumniczer Sandor in 1844.
E. Jules-Emile Péan in 1893.

50 Which one of the following is true regarding fundamental experimental microsurgical procedures?

A. Sun Lee's portocaval shunt operation in the rat was the first published procedure initiating the development of experimental microsurgery.
B. Kidney transplantation in a rat was the first published experimental microsurgical procedure.
C. Anastomoses of microvessels can be performed by cuff technique only.
D. Tissue transplantation can not be completed without vascular anastomoses.
E. None of the above is true.

Section 9 answers

History of plastic surgery

1   C.

China. The story of Wey Yong-Chi, the 18-year-old youth, whose lip was repaired by the Governor of Nanking's physician, was recorded by Morse in 1934 and by Wu LT Wong in 1936.

2   B.

Kernahan. Des Kernahan devised a classification with Richard B. Stark and described it in 1958. The primary palate is anterior to the incisive foramen and the secondary palate behind it.

3   A.

Clefts. Despite the title of the book, which does describe hernias, it is far reaching and covers many surgical subjects. Cleft lip repair is reported for the first time.

4   B.

McIndoe. Sir Archibald McIndoe used a skin graft passed through the penile shaft using a trocar, but the method had problems. Even if the graft survived, it contracted and stenosed. He had better luck with a similar technique for vaginal reconstruction, about which he delivered the Hunterian Oration - entitled: "Inlay grafting with special reference to obliterative conditions of the vagina", at The Royal College of Surgeons of England in 1940.

5 E.

Sir Harold Gillies described the full thickness skin graft. This statement is incorrect.

6 A.

Morestin. Hippolyte Morestin (1869-1919) was born on Martinique and became a military surgeon. His reputation for reconstructive surgery grew in WWI when he treated soldiers from the trenches at his unit in Paris. He was visited by Gillies who set up a similar hospital in Sidcup. He died of TB. The others are all French chefs, although there was also a plastic surgeon called Escoffier.

7 B.

Joseph. The famous Jacques Joseph (1885-1934) gained a reputation in Germany in WWI for his reconstructive skills and this probably saved him from Hitler's clutches. He worked in the famous Berlin Orthopaedic Unit of Professor Wolff and was "sacked from one post by performing a bat ear operation". His fame comes from his skill in rhinoplasty and his instruments are now in the Archive of the British Association of Plastic, Reconstructive and Aesthetic Surgeons (BAPRAS) at The Royal College of Surgeons of England.

8 B.

A urethral fistula. Astley Cooper and B. Travers used a scrotal flap to close a large urethral fistula in 1819.

9 C.

Browne. Denis Browne, the paediatric surgeon from Great Ormond Street Hospital, London, used a buried skin strip like Duplay had done in the previous century and then repaired the lateral skin over it by creating an everted suture line. Instead of tying the stitches he used beads and crushable lead stops. The repair was usually accompanied by a 'dorsal slit' along the length of the penis to relax the suture line and was protected by a perineal urethrostomy.

10 C.

Paré. Amboise Paré gives a beautiful description of chordee: "the band of the ligament of the yarde is too short so that the yarde cannot become straight and is turned downwards; in these cases the generation of children is hindered, because the seed cannot be passed directly and plentifully into the wombe." Therefore, this ligament must be removed with much dexterity.

11 D.

Voltaire. Of these authors, Samuel Butler (1612-1680) included a passage in his satirical poem Hudibras, while Voltaire wrote caustically about Tagliacozzi in 1785.

12 E.

Cowasjee. Cowasjee was a bullock cart driver in the service of the British East Indian Company army in the war with Tipu Sultan in 1792. He had his hand and nose cut off as punishment and the famous report of the reconstruction appeared in the *Gentleman's Magazine* of 1794.

References

1. PJ Sykes, IS Whitaker, K Shokrollahi. Another Barak from earlier times: elucidating the origins of rhinoplasty and solving the 'BL' mystery. *Ann Plast Surg* 2009; 63(1): 2-5.

13 B.

Carpue. After years of research and practice on cadavers, Joseph Constantine Carpue, an Englishman with Spanish ancestors, was so enthused by the 'BL' letter that he performed two successful reconstructions and reported his results in 1816.

14 D.

Padget. Padget's drum dermatome was designed to cut thick grafts in large square sheets. The others invented their own version of the guarded, variable-depth free graft knife following the one introduced by Humby.

15 B.

Paré. "Je le pansai et Dieu le guérit" is inscribed on his statue. He revolutionised the treatment of wounds by stopping the practice of cauterisation with hot iron. He also served as the surgeon to Kings of France.

16 A.

800-600 BC. There is considerable debate about his place and date of birth among Indian scholars but the evidence points to the earliest of these dates.

17 B.

Albucasis. He was born in the Moorish city of Cordoba in 936 and died in 1013. His encyclopedic work meaning *The Method*, focusing on medicine and surgery, heralded the rebirth of surgery after the fall of Rome.

18 C.

Galen. Cladius Galen (131-201 AD) was an advisor to three Roman Emperors and wrote over 100 texts. He was the undisputed authority for physicians and philosophers for centuries until his teachings were challenged in the 13th century by Theoderic of Cervia and Henri de Mondeville.

19 E.

Arabs. Cauterisation was known to all these races, but it was the Arabs who "practically set aside the knife" (Garrison 1912).

20 D.

Hippocrates. The maxim "First do no harm", is attributed to Hippocrates (ca. 460-355 BC) from Greece.

21 C.

Arabs. Much of the teaching and writings from classical times were lost during the Middle Ages only being preserved to some degree in the monasteries, but the Nestorians - who are said to have inherited part of the Great Library of Alexandria, established medical teaching in Arabia and translated classical works, such as those of Galen.

22 D.

Versalius. The beautifully illustrated book on anatomy was written by Andrea Versalius (1514-1564) who was born in the Belgian town of Wesen, but worked for most of his life at the University of Padua.

23 A.

Bologna. Being one of the first surgeons to attend university, he was born in Bologna; he worked there all his life and gained a doctorate before taking up anatomy and surgery.

24 C.

1597. The official Bindoni edition was printed in Venice in 1597 and was copied in a pirated version the same year. Tagliacozzi died shortly after its publication in 1599.

25 A.

Mercurialis. In 1586 Tagliacozzi wrote to the influential Mercurialis. He had visited Bologna to see the technique and wrote about nasal reconstruction in Italy in *De Decoratione Liber* published in 1585. The letter gave details of Tagliacozzi's further experience and was published in its entirety in the second edition of Mercurialis in 1587.

26 B.

Gnudi and Webster. In 1950, Martha Teach Gnudi, an academic, and Jerome Pierce Webster, a plastic surgeon who worked in Italy in WWII, wrote *The Life and Times of Gaspare Tagliacozzi, Surgeon of Bologna: 1545-1599*. The Herbert Reicher (New York) publication is a fascinating read and includes a documented study of the scientific and cultural life of Bologna in the 16th century.

27 A.

Zeis. The German surgeon and author of the first plastic surgery textbook, Eduard Zeis stated that the British had occupied India for almost two centuries, but had failed to inform the Western World about the Indian method of nasal reconstruction.

28 D.

All of these. Charles Bell wrote about these subjects. He was the brother of the surgeon John Bell.

29 A.

Gillies. In WWI, Major Harold Delft Gillies used a tube pedicle to reconstruct the face of able seaman Vicarage at Queen Mary's Hospital, Sidcup, in 1917. Unbeknownst to him a Russian ophthalmologist, Vladimir Filatov of Odessa, had used a small tube of skin from the neck to reconstruct the eyelid. This event was published in Russian in 1917. Aymard, a South African surgeon working at Sidcup, claimed to have been the first to use a tube pedicle and wrote up the procedure before Gillies in the *Lancet* in 1917. In fact, the theatre records show that Gillies did the operation on Vicarage some days before Aymard, who was present at the operation.

30 C.

Paré. He designed a prosthesis to replace a missing nose. The others all reconstructed noses.

31 C.

Baronio. Following his experiments using grafts on animals, mainly using the backs of rams, Giuseppe Baronio wrote *Degli Innesti Animale* in 1804. He demonstrated their feasibility and clarified several biological aspects of the method.

32 C.

India. Henri M Dutrochet wrote in 1817 that his brother-in-law had witnessed the procedure in India: "prior to cutting a graft from the buttock the skin was beaten vigorously with a slipper until this produced considerable swelling." Dutrochet discovered cell physiology and the process of osmosis. Tom Gibson of Glasgow wrote about the method in 1961.

33 C.

Thiersch. Carl Thiersch (1822-1895), from Munich, used very thin grafts. He experimented on the leg of a soldier who was about to have his limb amputated and made observations on the macroscopic and microscopic changes in these grafts on the limb once removed. He used a special razor to cut these very thin grafts which represented a shift in the prevalent method of thick grafting.

34 A.

Vincent van Gogh.

35 C.

Reverdin. Jacques Louis Reverdin (1842-1929) studied at Hôpital Necker in Paris. Like many surgeons of the day, he gained valuable experience in the Franco-Prussian War treating wounds and amputation stumps with his pinch grafts. After observing Reverdin's method, George Pollock returned to England where these grafts were called Pollock grafts. George Lawson then used larger, full thickness 'four-penny' grafts to cover all the surface of a granulating wound.

36 C.

Gibson. Tom Gibson of Glasgow worked on large numbers of burn victims from WWII and observed that although homografts survived for around 2 weeks, if the same donor was used a second time they were rejected immediately. This led to the seminal work carried out with Medawar from Oxford, which formed the basis for the immune response.

37 A.

Medawar. In 1942, Peter Medawar from Oxford worked with Tom Gibson at the Glasgow Royal Infirmary where large numbers of burn victims from WWII were treated with skin grafts. His work on the immune response to 'none-self' transplants led to the Nobel Prize shared with MacFarlane Burnett in 1960.

38 C.

Lawson. George Lawson (1831-1903) reported his experience with full thickness grafts to the Clinical Society of London in 1871 (a year after Reverdin's pinch grafts). They were about the size of a four-penny piece. He served as a surgeon in the Crimea where he survived severe illness. On his return, he specialised in ophthalmic surgery.

39 C.

They were ophthalmologists. They both worked as military surgeons in different campaigns, but they shared the specialty of ophthalmology.

40 D.

Blair and Barret-Brown. Vilray Papin Blair and James Barret-Brown from the Department of Medicine at Washington University reported on the use of large split skin grafts of intermediate thickness in 1929.

41 D.

All of these. Graham Humby devised his graft knife while at Great Ormond Street Hospital before he moved to Sydney.

42 A.

Lanz. The Swiss, Otto Lanz (1865-1935), introduced a simple instrument to mesh grafts in 1908 so as to halve the size of the donor site. The quote is by McDowell.

43 B.

Franco. Pierre Franco operated and wrote *Traites des Hernies* in 1561.

44 B.

Stephenson. One of Roux's earliest patients was a Canadian medical student, John Stephenson, who studied in Edinburgh before going to Paris. He reported his experience in 1820 at the University of Edinburgh and wrote a thesis on the subject.

45 A.

Thiersch.

46 C.

von Graefe. The two surgeons argued over who was the first to repair the cleft palate so vigorously that it became an issue of national honour. von Graefe presented his achievement in a brief paper to the Medical Society of Berlin and this was reported in a little known local publication with a small circulation in 1816. His main publication appeared in 1817. Believing sincerely that he had been the first, Roux reported the details of a similar operation in 1819.

47 E.

Galen.

48 B.

Phemister. Dallas B. Phemister published his paper on the fate of transplanted bone in 1914 and it appeared to resolve the debate about whether or not it was necessary to include periosteum. He showed that many small pieces of bone alone survived better and produced more bone than a single large piece due to improved vascularisation.

49 C.

Iginio Tansini in 1896. The latissimus dorsi myocutaneous flap procedure was firstly described by the Italian pioneer surgeon Iginio Tansini (1855-1943) in 1896. The flap procedure was combined with a radical mastectomy and was used to close the chest wall defect. The radical mastectomy was developed and first performed by William Stewart Halsted (1852-1922) in 1882.

Lumniczer Sandor (1821-1892) published a dissertation on plastic surgery in Hungarian in 1844 (first Hungarian plastic surgery book). Jules-Emile Péan (1830-1898), leader French surgeon of the era, performed a shoulder reconstruction using total joint arthroplasty in 1893. Alexis Carrel (1873-1944) was awarded the Nobel Prize in 1912 for new techniques in vascular sutures and pioneering work in transplantology and thoracic surgery.

References

1. Tansini I. Nuovo processo per l'amputazione della mammaella perla cancre. *Reforma Medica* 1896; 12: 3.
2. Maxwell G. Iginio Tansini and the origin of the latissimus dorsi musculocutaneous flap. *Plast Reconstr Surg* 1980; 65: 686-92.

50 A.

Sun Lee's portocaval shunt operation in the rat was the first published procedure initiating the development of experimental microsurgery. The end-to-side portocaval shunt was perfected in the rat by Dr. Sun Lee (Sil

Heung Lee) in 1958, published in 1961. It was the beginning of experimental microsurgery and opened the way to perform various organ and tissue transplantation procedures in rats and mice using advanced microsurgical techniques. Dr. Bernard Fisher (University of Pittsburg, USA) said in his book: "Do you know what you have done just now? You have opened an avenue to conduct allied physiological research, transplantation investigation..." Later Sun Lee developed and refined rat pancreatico-duodenum, liver, stomach, spleen, and heart-lung transplants.

References

1.   Lee SH, Fisher B. Portacaval shunt in the rat. *Surgery* 1961; 50: 668-72.

2.   Zhong R. 'Father' of experimental microsurgery: Dr. Sun Lee. *Microsurgery* 2003; 23: 412-3.